LASERS
IN
SKIN
DISEASE

Published Volumes

Proportions of the Aesthetic Face
Powell and Humphreys

Facial Reconstruction with Local and Regional Flaps
Becker

Rhinoplasty: Emphasizing the External Approach
Anderson and Ries

Surgery of the Mandible
Bailey and Holt

Forthcoming Volumes

Dermabrasion and Chemical Peels
McCullough and Langsdon

Free Flap Reconstruction in Head and Neck Surgery
Panje and Moran

Hair Rejuvenation
Fleming and Mayer

Rhinoplasty
Simons

Medicolegal Issues in Facial Plastic Surgery
Thomas and Thomas

The American Academy of Facial Plastic and Reconstructive Surgery

Series Editor: James D. Smith, M.D.

LASERS IN SKIN DISEASE

Ronald G. Wheeland, M.D., F.A.C.P.
Associate Professsor
Chief, Mohs and Laser Surgery
Department of Dermatology
University of California
Davis Medical Center
Sacramento, California

1988
Thieme Medical Publishers, Inc.
Georg Thieme Verlag, Stuttgart · New York

Thieme Medical Publishers, Inc.
381 Park Avenue South
New York, New York 10016

Series sponsored by the educational committee of The American Academy of Facial Plastic and Reconstructive Surgery.

LASERS IN SKIN DISEASE
Ronald G. Wheeland

Library of Congress Cataloging in Publication Data

Wheeland, Ronald G.
   Lasers in skin disease.

   (The American Academy of Facial Plastic and Reconstructive Surgery)
   Includes index.
   1. Lasers—Therapeutic use. 2. Skin—Diseases—Treatment. I. Title. II. Series: American Academy of Facial Plastic and Reconstructive Surgery (Series) [DNLM: 1. Laser Surgery. 2. Skin Diseases—surgery. WR 650 W561L]
RL120.L37W47   1988   616.5′0631   87-26695

Printed in the United States of America.

TMP ISBN 0-86577-271-1
GTV ISBN 3-13-713401-3

TMP (series) 0-86577-135-5
GTV (series) 3-13-656501-0

This book is dedicated to my loving and understanding wife, Martha Mansur Wheeland; my fantastic, energetic, and stimulating sons, Chris, Matt, and Jeff; and my caring parents, George P. and Beulah M. Wheeland, all of whom offered me their continuous support and encouragement, not only during the creation of this text, but also throughout my medical career. Without their loving concern and wise counsel, this text would not have been possible.

Acknowledgments

My initial introduction and primary stimulus to become interested in surgery came rather early in my medical training from the dean of my medical school, Dr. Merlin K. DuVal, at the University of Arizona. He stimulated me to think, question, reason, and not blindly accept the prevalent surgical dogma. The importance of him challenging me to develop an inquiring mind was, of course, essential for my later acceptance and usage of laser technology. The role he has played in my career has been substantial.

The next important step in my developmental process came from my first partner, Dr. Patrick E. Watson of Missoula, Montana, who through his meticulous technique and caring demeanor taught me many valuable surgical and nonsurgical skills. Later, my chairman at the University of Oklahoma, Dr. Mark Allen Everett, was sympathetic to my proposal of developing a laser surgical service and was extremely supportive in helping me acquire those skills which have led me to my current position today.

Every laser surgeon owes a special debt of thanks to Dr. Leon Goldman who is considered to be the "godfather" of laser medicine and surgery, for it was he who had the vision of recognizing the potential offered by the new technology of lasers to the fields of medicine and surgery. His initial nurturing and enthusiastic development of treatment protocols and techniques, as well as his continued involvement even today, underscores the valuable role he has played in the evolutionary process of laser surgery.

Lastly, I am deeply grateful for having had the opportunity to work with the superb equipment, and excellent nursing and technical staff provided by both the Cleveland Clinic Foundation and University of California, Davis Medical Center. These individuals and organizations have allowed me to continue my investigations over the past five years and are jointly responsible for numerous advances made in the clinical treatment of a variety of cutaneous disorders.

Preface

Over the 26 years since their initial introduction, laser technology has provided the surgeon with an effective form of treatment for a large variety of disorders of both skin and internal organs. Today, the laser has become an almost universally accepted instrument for most medical and surgical specialties. While some specialties such as ophthalmology, dermatology, and otolaryngology currently rely heavily on various laser systems in the daily practice of medicine, the potential of the laser has not been fully recognized by all specialties. It is certain, however, that with additional improvements as well as the development of new instruments, the role of the medical laser will certainly expand tremendously in the very near future.

In the treatment of disorders of the skin and mucous membranes, laser technology has provided an effective form of treatment for lesions of the head and neck for which no therapy or only very poor forms of therapy previously existed. The proper usage of lasers in the treatment of human disease includes knowing when use of the laser is appropriate as well as when *not* to use the laser. Sadly, the trend has been in certain specialties for some laser surgeons to treat every disease with the laser regardless of the appropriateness of that treatment. It is reminiscent of the adage, "If all you have is a hammer, then everything begins to look like a nail."

It is for this reason that a complete understanding of the basic properties of the common lasers in use today for the treatment of skin and mucous membrane disorders and how they can be most effectively utilized in various clinical settings is essential. The goal of this text is to describe the various uses of the argon and carbon dioxide lasers in various clinical settings and provide the practitioner with a basic understanding of the way lasers are designed and interact with tissue. In this way, the full potential of these exciting tools may be realized in the future.

Foreword

Otolaryngologic doctors years ago were interested in laser surgery of extensive facial and oral lesions. These lesions were vascular types and neoplasms. With dermatologists, cooperative studies were done with Mohs-controlled surgery to evaluate the depth and efficacy of laser surgery.

The initial oral lesions treated were leukoplakia, angiomas, and tumors before the development of laser endoscopy for laryngeal papillomas and malignancies. The lasers used were the ruby laser and later, the carbon dioxide laser. From a historical aspect, Bellina, a pioneer laser gynecologist, derived his interest and development from the laser ear, nose, and throat applications. The laser otolaryngologic applications led to the development of laser plastic surgery.

Leon Goldman, M.D.
Professor Emeritus Dermatology
College of Medicine
University of Cincinnati
Director, Laser Research Laboratory
Medical Director, Laser Treatment Center
Cincinnati, Ohio

Contents

LASERS
IN
SKIN
DISEASE

1 Fundamental Laser Physics for the Surgeon and Laser-Tissue Interaction

Lasers in their simplest form are merely pure sources of light. Of course, light has been used in the treatment of a variety of diseases for thousands of years, but the laser is an extremely complex system composed of radiant energy in the form of photons and waves. This system is organized according to the size of the waves of the various sources of energy into the electromagnetic spectrum (Table 1). The distance between two successive crests determines the wavelength of the light energy. This, in turn, accounts for the color of visible light or the portion of the electromagnetic spectrum to which the energy source is assigned its position. The wavelength and frequency are two factors that are inversely related to one another so that shorter wavelengths of light have a higher frequency and greater energy than the longer wavelengths of light.

All forms of laser energy represent different types of light. In fact, the word laser is an acronym which stands for Light Amplification by the Stimulated Emission of Radiation. Thus, a laser is not only a surgical tool, but also a physical process resulting from the amplification of energy. The first historical reference to the use of light energy was described in the fictional book, "War of the Worlds," written by H.G. Wells in 1896. In this book, the Martian aliens utilize a "heat ray" to destroy the English villages. However, it wasn't until 1916 that Albert Einstein actually developed the theoretical concept of the laser.

While the last word in the acronym LASER, radiation, is a cause of some concern to both patients and physicians alike, most sources of medical and surgical laser energy available today do not employ ionizing radiation. Consequently, laser radiation is not associated with the same risks that are inherent with the high energy forms of ionizing radiation used in the therapeutic management of internal malignancies.

The first actual stimulated emission of radiation occured in 1954 in the microwave portion of the electromagnetic spectrum. This instrument known as a MASER which stands for Microwave Amplification by the Stimulated Emission of Radiation, was developed by Townes. The first truly functional laser, the ruby laser, was developed in 1960 by Theodore Maiman.

The three lasers that are crucial to this text were also developed in the relatively recent past. The helium-neon (HeNe) was developed in 1962 by workers at Bell Laboratories and, while this laser has little or no biologic activity, it is of tremendous usefulness to the carbon dioxide laser system since this red light serves as an aiming beam for the accurate positioning of the invisible carbon dioxide laser energy. This laser has also found wide acceptance as a pointing device in large lectures halls and conferences.

Developed as the argon ion laser in 1964 by Bridges, the argon laser has now been extensively used in the treatment of a number of cutaneous and mucous membrane disorders and has been the mainstay of treatment for a variety of vascular conditions. In 1964, the carbon dioxide laser was developed and has, now over the intervening 23 years, proven to be the most useful laser available for the majority of medical and surgical specialities. Since 1964, a number of other laser systems have been developed which have found selective usefulness in only certain specialities. One example is the neodymium:YAG (Nd:YAG) laser which has been used extensively in gastroenterology, but has been of only limited usefulness in the treatment of cutaneous disorders because of the diffuse effects of this energy source. A number of other laser systems are currently on the physicists optical bench (Table 2) and are certain to provide a variety of new and useful therapeutic options for a number of cutaneous and internal diseases in the future.

THE CREATION OF LASER LIGHT

In order to understand how laser energy is created, it is beneficial to review some basic physical

Table I. The Electromagnetic Spectrum

Type of Radiation	Wavelength
Cosmic	0.00001 nm
X-ray	0.1 nm
Ultraviolet	10 nm to 100nm
Visible	400 nm to 700nm
violet	430 nm
blue	490 nm
green	530 nm
yellow	577 nm
orange	590 nm
red	630 nm
Infrared	770 nm to 12,000 nm
near	1,000 nm
mid	10,000 nm
far	12,000 nm
Microwave	1.0 cm
Television and FM radio	100 cm
AM radio	10,000 cm

Table 2. Medical Laser Systems

Argon	488–514 nm
Carbon dioxide	10,600 nm
Dye (rhodamine G)	544, 577, 633 nm
Nd:YAG	1,064 nm
Doubled-YAG	532 nm
Ruby	694 nm
Helium-neon	632.8 nm
Copper vapor	510, 540, 578, 620, 650, 690 nm
Gallium-arsenide	904 nm
Gold head vapor	630 nm
Helium-cadmiun	325–441 nm
Krypton ion	458, 568, 647 nm
Nitrogen	337 nm
Excimer	193, 248, 308, 351 nm
Xenon-fluoride	351 nm

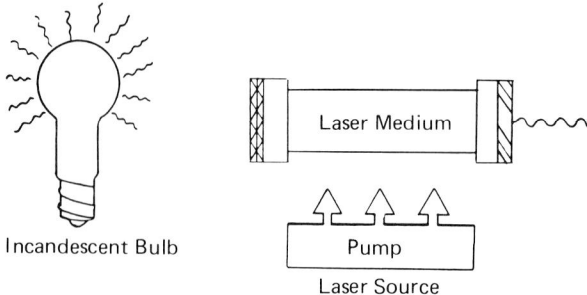

Figure 1. This schematic demonstrates the difference between incoherent light from an incandescent light bulb and coherent light from a laser light source.

principles. An atom is the smallest, complete amount of any substance and is composed of a single nucleus containing positive charged particles, protons, surrounded by negative-charged particles, electrons, which orbit the central nucleus at precisely defined energy levels and distances from the nucleus. The electons move continuously from their resting energy levels to excited energy levels when the atom absorbs energy. The outer orbits have higher energy and when an electron is in this position, the atom becomes unstable. As a consequence, the electron rapidly returns to its resting energy position around the nucleus and at the same time releases a small amount of energy known as a photon.

In a natural state, this energy release is random and without order and occurs spontaneously in a fraction of a second. This type of energy release is typified by what occurs when an incandescent light bulb is turned on and the light source is known as incoherent light. This released energy is incoherent since it occurs in all directions (Fig. 1). The motion of one photon of light is completely unrelated to any other photons of light that are released from other energy orbits. That is, these photons are moving at different rates of speed and in different directions.

In order to create laser energy, the atoms within the laser chamber must exist in their higher unstable energy configurations, a condition which is known as population inversion. This is obtained in most medical laser systems by energizing the laser chamber with electricity. The electricity energizes an atom and causes the electrons to assume an unstable, high-energy, orbital configuration. When this situation occurs, if a photon of energy strikes an excited atom, the return of the stimulated electron to its resting energy configuration is stimulated. This stimulation results in two photons of energy released from the atom at precisely the same moment; they then travel together in the same direction and at the same rate of speed with one another. This is the first step in the creation of a laser beam.

LASER COMPONENTS

Typically, all medical lasers are composed of the same four components. The first of these is an optical cavity or resonating tube which surrounds a laser medium (Fig. 2). The laser medium typically is formed from a solid, liquid, or

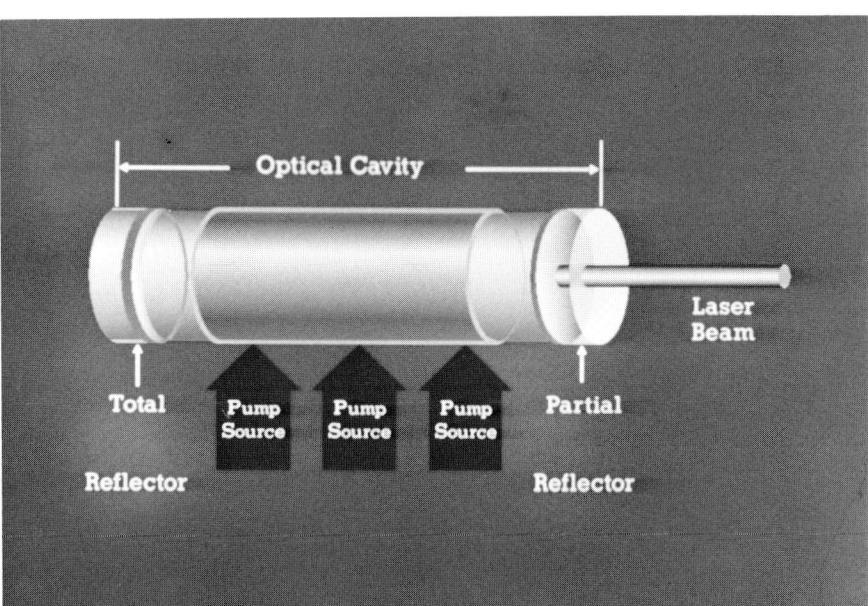

Figure 2. A schematic showing the optical cavity with totally reflecting mirrored end and partially reflecting mirrored end through which the laser beam is emitted. The energizing source is known as the pump.

gas and gives the name to the laser system itself. Within the optical cavity, the excitation process occurs when an external source of energy, known as the pump, delivers energy to the system. This excitation mechanism results in the absorption of energy by the contained atoms causing the creation of population inversion. Most of the laser systems in medical use today employ either direct electrical current, radiofrequency, or rarely, light for the pump, while only a few lasers employ a chemical reaction to create population inversion.

The fourth and final component of all lasers is the delivery system. For the argon laser, this consists of a fiber, since fiberoptics are capable of delivering laser energy of most visible wavelengths of light. They are also under investigation for delivery of invisible laser energy sources such as the Nd:YAG and carbon dioxide lasers. In the meantime, while this developmental process is occurring, carbon dioxide laser energy is generally delivered to the target tissue by means of articulated, angled-mirrored joints. A recent FDA-approved innovation is the flexible, hollow fiber which permits the carbon dioxide laser energy to be delivered in a curved line without the use of articulating-mirrored joints.

CHARACTERISTICS OF LASER LIGHT

Laser energy is different from all natural forms of light energy in three very important ways.

First, laser energy is coherent which means the waves of energy released from a laser chamber travel through space and time oriented with one another (Fig. 3). Secondly, the laser light is collimated, which means, that from its emission point the beam of energy does not diverge as it travels through space even over very long distances. This is due to the parallel transmission of laser light and permits extremely accurate delivery of laser energy to a target. Lastly, laser energy is monochromatic, which means that for visible laser energy sources, the light is of a single color. For invisible laser energy sources, the energy is released as a single wavelength or narrow band of wavelengths. While this statement is made, in truth, a single source of laser energy may actually be composed of multiple wavelengths that are relatively close to one another and for practical

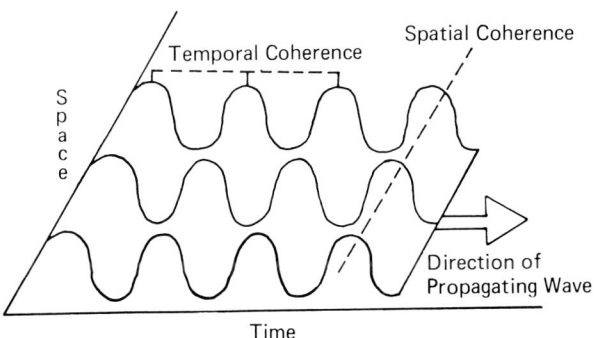

Figure 3. As laser energy moves through space, it is coherent both temporally and spatially as it is propagated.

purposes can be viewed as a single wavelength of light. The argon laser is one example of this phenomenon since there are no fewer than six peaks of laser energy released by the argon laser varying from 488 to 514 nm. On the other hand, the carbon dioxide laser has almost total energy release at 10,600 nm.

LASER DESIGN

Within the optical cavity, amplification of light occurs through the absorption of externally applied energy. Optical cavities can be viewed as tubular structures having mirrors on both ends. One of these mirrored ends has a small perforation that allows release of a small quantity of laser energy (Fig. 2). Photons of laser energy are reflected back and forth many times between the two ends of the mirrored optical cavity. As each transit occurs, there is a geometric progression in the energy being created as one photon strikes an energized atom releasing two photons which, in turn, strikes two additional energized atoms releasing four photons and so forth until a tremendous amplification of the energy within the optical cavity occurs.

In spite of this fact, lasers are intrinsically inefficient. The argon laser, for example, has an efficiency of 0.1% and much of the external energy supplied by direct electrical current is lost from this laser as waste heat. The carbon dioxide laser, by comparision, is a much more efficient laser with an efficiency of 10% to 15%. However, as can be quickly seen, even the carbon dioxide laser will have a tremendous amount of energy lost as waste heat. This may be important in the clinical setting since the argon laser may require special plumbing to permit water cooling of the the laser and prevent overheating of the equipment, the patient, and the operating suite. Carbon dioxide lasers, on the other hand, are generally air-cooled to rid the system of the waste heat that is generated. However, special air conditioning or ventilation may be required in the carbon dioxide laser operating suite to prevent overheating of the physician, the patient, or the equipment.

Once the laser beam has been generated and is emitted from the optical cavity through the small perforation in the partially reflective mirror, it can be delivered to the target and focused by a standard lens of predetermined focal length. This focal length is usually determined by the manufacture of the laser equipment, but in certain circumstances, a variety of different focal lengths

may be available to allow the surgeon the greatest flexibility in application of laser energy to a specific medical condition or problem.

BIOLOGIC EFFECTS OF LASER TISSUE INTERACTION

Once the beam of laser energy has been released from the optical cavity, in order to properly employ the laser energy in a given clinical situation, several additional concepts must be understood to achieve a given biologic effect. First, in order to appropriately select the best laser system to treat a given condition, it must be understood that various lasers have different effects on living tissue. These effects are generally related to the wavelength of light being emitted by the laser.

The interaction of laser light with living tissue is also dependent upon the optical characteristics of the target itself. If a given form of laser energy is completely transmitted through a tissue without any absorption, no biologic effect will occur. Likewise, if laser energy is reflected from the surface of a biologic tissue, there will also be no interaction and no biologic effect will occur. If absorption of laser energy by the living tissue is relatively imprecise and nonspecific, the effects on that tissue will also be imprecise as the energy is scattered.

However, the laser surgeon would ideally like to have a specific interaction of emitted laser energy through selective absorption within the target. For the carbon dioxide laser, this specific interaction occurs between intracellular or ex-

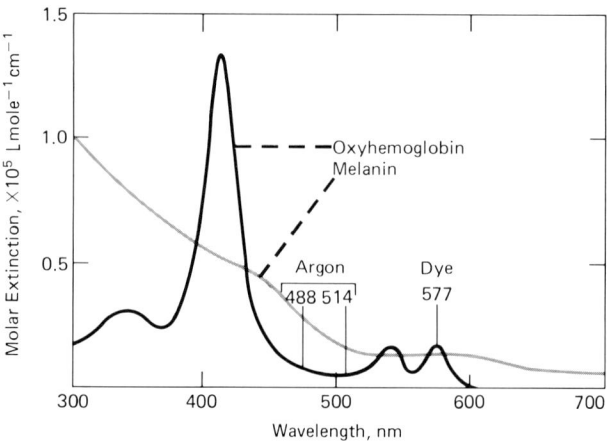

Figure 4. Absorption spectra of hemoglobin and melanin with the emission spectra of the argon and dye lasers superimposed.

tracellular water and the carbon dioxide laser energy. For the argon laser (Fig. 4), this specific absorption occurs between the hemoglobin and melanin content of the target and the blue-green argon laser light. In both of these situations, since the absorption of the emitted laser energy is precisely absorbed by one of the components of the target, a relatively precise and selective effect can be achieved. This principle allows the laser surgeon to select the best laser light source from a variety of different wavelengths to most precisely treat a given disorder or condition.

Irradiance

When a beginning laser surgeon reviews the literature in an attempt to understand how a more experienced laser surgeon has treated a given condition, it is important to be able to employ the same parameters even on different laser equipment in order to achieve the same beneficial effects. The irradiance, also known as power density, determines the ability of a given laser to incise, vaporize, or coagulate tissues. This term is generally expressed in watts/cm^2 and its calculation is based on the formula:

$$\frac{\text{Irradiance}}{(\text{Watts/cm}^2)} = \frac{\text{Laser output (watts)} \times 100}{\pi \times \text{radius}^2 \text{ (of the laser beam)}}$$

Some typical irradiances for laser beams of standard size and power settings are as follows:

Beam Diameter

Power (Watts)	0.2 mm	0.5 mm	1.0 mm	2.0 mm
5	15,920	2,550	640	160
10	31,830	5,090	1,270	320
15	47,700	7,640	1,910	480
20	63,700	10,190	2,550	640

By understanding the concept and calculations of irradiance, two surgeons can use different lasers, manufactured by different companies and still get equivalent results by employing proper beam size and energy levels to yield equal irradiances.

Energy Fluence

The second term used to describe the quality and quantity of laser energy delivered to a target tissue is energy fluence. This is the amount of energy delivered to a given unit area of tissue for a single pulse. This calculation is based on the formula:

$$\frac{\text{Energy fluence}}{(\text{joules/cm}^2)} = \frac{\text{Laser output (watts)} \times \text{exposure (sec)}}{\pi \times \text{radius}^2 \text{ (of the laser beam)}}$$

By knowing the amount of energy delivered for a single pulse, the energy characteristics of the laser beam can be constantly maintained at the same level throughout a series of laser treatments as is required for a large lesion such as a portwine stain.

A third concept that is sometimes used to describe the laser parameters is that of spatial average energy fluence which averages the total amount of energy delivered to a given treatment area. This term is sometimes abbreviated SAEF and its calculation is based on the following formula:

$$\text{SAEF} = \frac{\text{Laser output (watts)} \times \text{pulse number} \times \text{exposure time (sec)}}{\text{size of the treated area (cm}^2)}$$

By understanding this term, it is possible to standardize treatment parameters from one instrument or laser facility to another and still obtain similar effects.

Biologic Effects

In order for any form of laser energy to cause a given effect in a target tissue, it must first be absorbed. To properly select the most ideal laser system to treat a cutaneous or mucous membrane condition or disorder, the surgeon must understand how laser energy can produce a specific biologic effect in tissue. The interaction of light with living tissue is dependent upon the wavelength of the laser system producing the light energy as well as the optical characteristics of the target itself.

The two most commonly used lasers in the treatment of cutaneous disorders create their effect in tissue largely by the transformation of light energy into thermal energy. For the argon laser, this effect is relatively selective in nature due to the absorption of the blue-green argon laser light by the two main chromophores of the skin, hemoglobin and melanin. For the carbon dioxide laser, this absorption is by intracellular or extracellular water. Through this specific interaction with the blue-green light energy, heating of blood-filled vascular channels or pigmented tissue will occur following contact with argon laser energy resulting in thermal injury and subsequent removal by phagocytosis. Similarly, the carbon dioxide laser energy absorption results in instantaneous conversion of intracellular or extracellular water to steam and smoke with minimal conduction of thermal energy into the adjacent tissue.

COMMON LASER TERMS

Absorption   The transformation of radiant energy to another form of energy, usually heat, through the specific interaction with matter.

Coherence   Energy wave forms travel in phase with one another through time and space.

Collimation   All energy wave forms are emitted in parallel fashion and can be transmitted through space without divergence or convergence.

Electromagnetic radiation   A complex system of radiant energy that consists of waves and energy bundles organized according to the length of the propagating wave.

Energy   The product of time (seconds) and power (watts) which is expressed in joules.

Focus   The exact point at which laser energy being emitted from an optical cavity is at its peak power; this point can be modified by the interpositional placement of lenses having different focal lengths.

Irradiance (power density)   The quotient of an incident laser energy beam on a unit surface area which is expressed as watts/cm².

Joule   A unit of energy which is equal to one watt-second.

Laser   An instrument that is capable of generating a beam of light having a single color or wavelength which is both highly coherent and collimated; also an acronym which stands for Light Amplification by the Stimulated Emission of Radiation.

Lasing Medium   A material contained within an optical cavity that may be of solid, gaseous, or liquid nature and is capable of producing a laser light source by the stimulated transition of unstable, high-energy electrons from outer orbits to more stable, low-energy, inner orbits through the release of collimated, coherent, monochromatic light.

Meter   A unit of length based on the spectrum of krypton-86; typically subdivided into mm (10^{-3} meters), micrometers (10^{-6} meters), and nanometers (10^{-9} meters).

Monochromatic   A light energy having only one color or a narrow band of wavelengths.

Optically-pumped lasers   A laser where the excitation of orbital electrons is due to the absorption of light energy from some external source; this typically is another laser or a flashlamp.

Population inversion   The state present within the laser optical cavity in which more atoms of the laser medium exist in high, unstable energy configurations than in their normal, resting energy configurations.

Power   The rate at which energy is transmitted from a laser handpiece.

Power Density (irradiance)   The quotient of incident laser power on a unit surface area which is expressed as watts/cm².

Pump   The external source of energy that causes the development of population inversion within an optical cavity; this may be in the form of direct electrical energy, optical energy, radiofrequency, or rarely, chemical excitation.

Reflection   An incident laser beam being diverted from the surface of its target without having the opportunity to interact with tissue.

Scatter   A nonspecific and diffuse effect that occurs when incident laser energy strikes a target tissue and is absorbed in a nonspecific broad pattern; this typically results in a zonal type of destruction with inadvertent injury to adjacent normal surrounding tissue.

Transmission   When an incident beam of laser energy passes completely through a target tissue resulting in no biologic effect since absorption of the laser energy by any given component of the target itself did not occur.

BIBLIOGRAPHY

Arndt KA, Noe JM: Lasers in dermatology. Arch Dermatol 118:293–295, 1982.

Fuller TA: The physics of surgical lasers. Lasers Surg Med 1:5–14, 1980.

Goldman L, Taylor A, Putnam T: New developments with the heavy metal vapor lasers for the dermatologist. J Dermatol Surg Oncol 13:163–165, 1987.

Wheeland RG, Walker NPJ: Lasers—25 years later. Internat J Dermatol 25:209–216, 1986.

2 The Argon Laser

The argon ion laser, most commonly referred to as the argon laser (Table 3), has been used extensively in the treatment of vascular disorders and pigmented conditions of the skin and mucous membranes for years. This laser light source is blue-green in color and has an emission spectrum between 488 and 514 nm. The reason this laser has been used extensively in these types of conditions is a function of this emission spectrum. Ideally, the laser surgeon would like to have the peak energy emission from any laser light source match exactly the peak absorption spectrum of a given target tissue. In this way, a precise and specific effect can be predicted.

If the emission spectrum for the argon laser (Figure 4) is examined and compared to the absorption spectrum of hemoglobin and melanin, one will find there is distinct overlap. Even though there is not an absolute match between the absorption and emission from these target tissue chromophores and the argon laser, it is sufficiently specific to result in a relative selective effect on these two types of tissue. Although some scatter of energy occurs within skin and mucous membranes following exposure to the argon laser light source, relative selectively is still present.

The argon laser energy is created when a high voltage electrical current is applied to the optical cavity containing argon gas. The emitted blue-green laser light can be transmitted efficiently along fiberoptics for some distance without much energy loss. The energy is delivered to the target tissue with a small pencil-like handpiece (Figure 5) from these rather large pieces of equipment (Figures 6 and 7). Advances in argon laser technology now permit a telescoping handpiece to be attached to the fiberoptics so that a laser beam of variable size can be employed without having to switch to a different size fiber from the optical cavity (Figure 8).

Even though this laser is used at relatively low irradiances, the amount of energy necessary to generate the argon laser beam is sufficiently high to require special wiring and water cooling in some cases. The efficiency of this laser is so low, on the order of 0.1%, that much of the energy applied to the system is lost as waste heat. Until recently, most argon lasers were water cooled and required modest water pressure for proper functioning. With current refinements, however, now air cooling is possible.

CLINICIAL USEFULNESS OF THE ARGON LASER

The main usefulness of the argon laser in the treatment of cutaneous and mucous membrane disorders has been in the photocoagulation of vascular, as well as pigmented lesions (Table 4). This is possible because of the relative specific absorption by the two main chromophores of the skin, melanin and hemoglobin, of the argon laser energy which is converted into heat. Through this interaction, the laser creates thermal injury in the cutaneous vasculature and pigment-containing cells while sparing the nonpigmented, normal, surrounding skin and soft tissue. The nature of this thermal injury and depth to which it occurs in the skin is dependent upon the quantity of the chromophore present within the tissue. The greater the quantity of these pigments within the target tissue, the more superficial the effects will be, since complete absorption will occur nearer the skin surface and, thus, limit the penetration of the argon laser energy.

The irradiance of the impacting beam and the time period it is in contact with tissue (energy fluence) also will determine the type of thermal injury that occurs in the target tissue. In general, the argon laser energy will penetrate to a depth of 1 to 2 mm before being completely absorbed by skin and mucous membranes. It is for this reason that the argon laser is not a beneficial form of treatment when the blood vessels are large or located in the deeper portions of the skin. In these situations, the more deeply penetrating Nd:YAG laser has been used with greater success. It must also be remembered that argon laser energy is scattered significantly in skin and mucous membranes. This scattering can decrease the specificity of the interaction with the target chromophore and result in nonspecific thermal injury of the adjacent tissue.

When treating patients having naturally dark skin color and significant melanin is present at the base of the epidermis or within the upper dermis, an inability of the argon laser energy to

Table 3. Physical Properties and Characteristics of the Argon Laser

Gas medium	Argon ion gas
Absorption pattern	Hemoglobin, melanin
Electromagnetic spectrum	Blue-green (visible light)
Wavelength	2 peaks at 488 nm and 514 nm
Type of emission	Continuous
Pumping energy	Electrical
Efficiency	0.1%
Method of delivery	Fiberoptics
Thermal conduction	Considerable
Soft-tissue destruction	Zonal
Coefficient of extinction	230 mm of water
Depth of penetration	1 – 1.5 mm of tissue
Amount of tissue scatter	Moderate (100 times greater than CO_2)
Power densities	
focused	10 to 200 watts/cm²
defocused	Cannot be operated in a defocused mode
Impact spot (beam diameter)	0.5 mm – 6 mm

penetrate through the melanin mass into the dermis may occur. Even in light-skinned individuals, there may be some absorption of argon laser energy by the superficial melanin pigmentation. The effect of this absorption may be immediate blistering or a popping sound at the time of argon laser treatment as the heat transferred to the epi-

dermis causes the upper layers of the epidermis and stratum corneum to expand rapidly and pop. This may also result in postoperative erythema and swelling caused by thermal damage to the superficial layers of the epidermis.

In light-skinned individuals, the result of this scatter of thermal energy by the target tissue may cause sufficient dermal heating to result in abnormal scar formation. If overt scarring is not seen, there may be sufficient textural change in the treated tissue to cause significant cosmetic disfigurement. In order to minimize the changes of adverse results, most argon laser surgeons will perform a small test site within a larger treatment zone and then permit healing to occur over a six- to 12-week interval to observe for possible abnormal scar formation or pigmentation that may compromise the final cosmetic result and make further laser treatment undesirable.

ANGIOMAS — PORTWINE STAIN BIRTHMARKS

There is no condition currently treated by the laser surgeon where the results can be more rewarding, both emotionally to the physician as well as cosmetically to the patient, as for the angioma or portwine stain. This condition was only very poorly treated prior to the development of laser technology and now most patients can expect to see significant improvement with argon laser photocoagulation. In fact, the laser surgeon

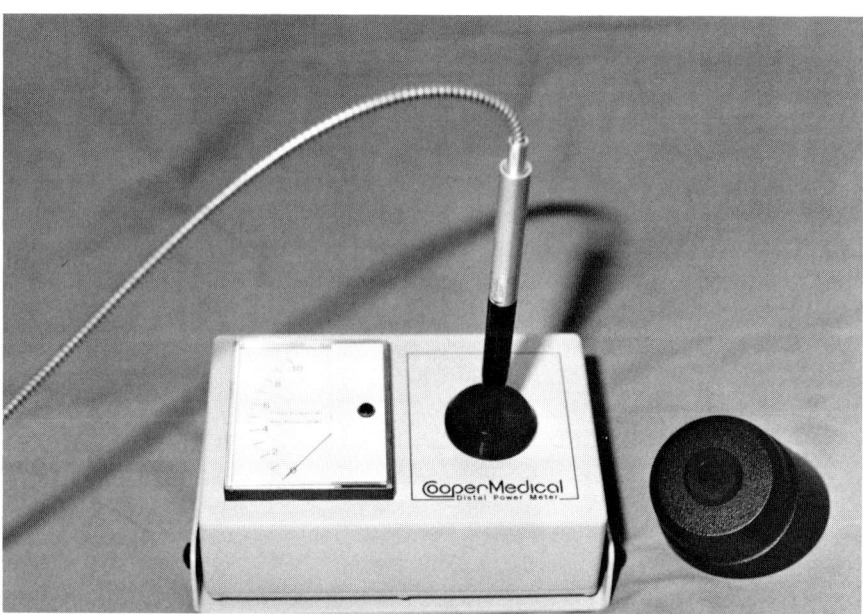

Figure 5. Fiberoptic extending from argon laser unit to pencil-like handpiece.

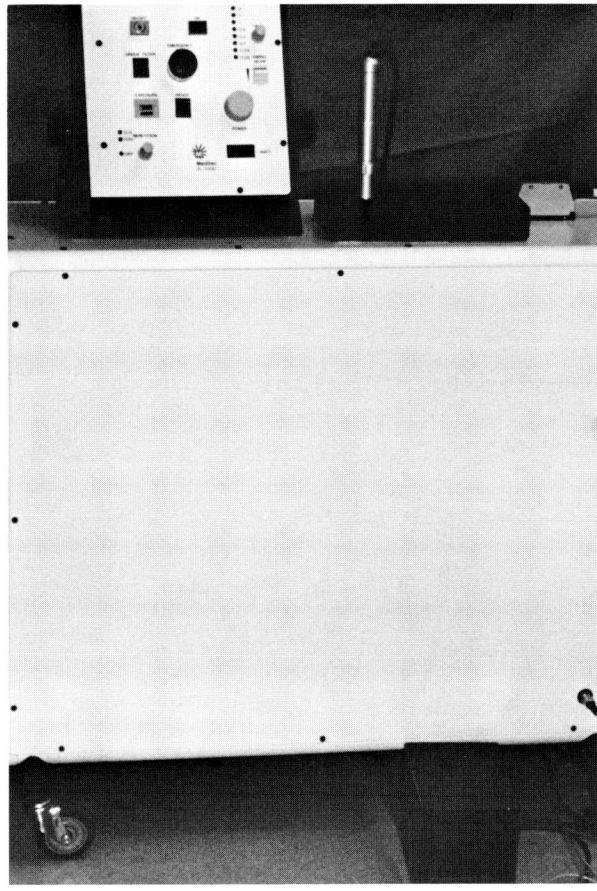

Figure 6. Argon laser with console mounted on top.

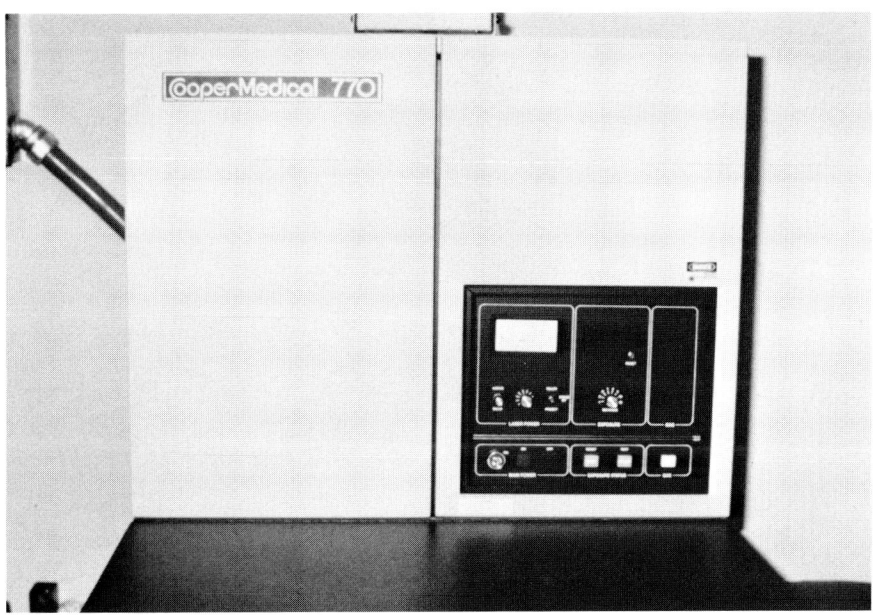

Figure 7. Argon laser with console mounted in the unit and also showing water-cooling tubing extending from the back of the unit.

Figure 8. Telescoping argon laser handpiece to give variable beam size.

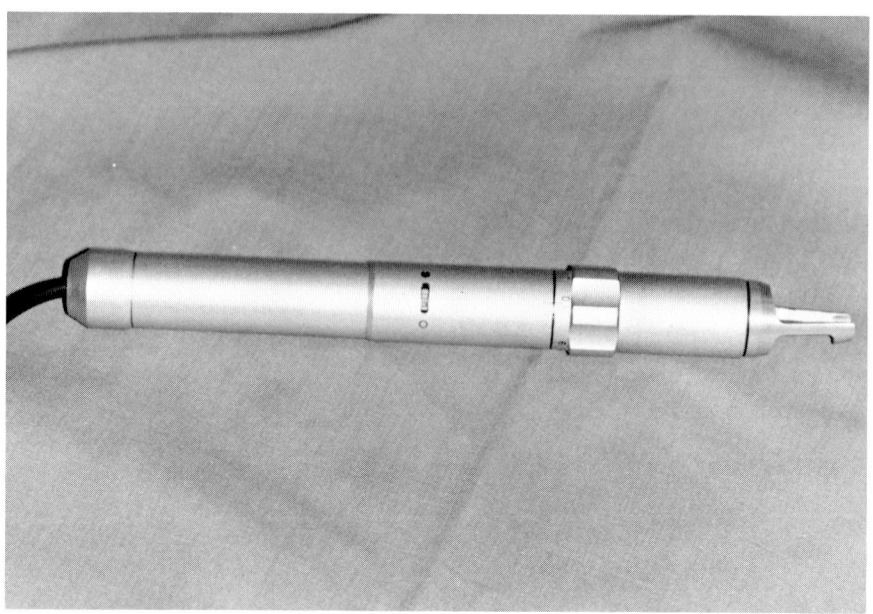

can predict that between 80% and 90% of patients suffering from superficial angiomas, without a deep or cavernous component, will obtain 70% to 80% lightening with argon laser phototherapy (Figures 9–12) (see color insert). This does not mean, however, that the laser surgeon can make the affected side of the face look like the unaffected side (Figures 13–16) and the individual degree of improvement is certainly dependent upon other factors such as the amount of color present prior to treatment and anatomic

Table 4. Clinical Applications of the Argon Laser

Vascular conditions
  Angioma serpiginosa
  Telangiectasia
    Spider angioma
    Acne rosacea (Rhinophyma)
    Solar
    Steroid induced
    Collagen-vascular disorders
    Hereditary hemorrhagic telangiectasia
  Portwine stain
  Venous lake
  Hemolymphangioma
  Carcinoidosis
  Senile (cherry) angioma
  Pyogenic granuloma
  Capillary hemangioma
  Angiokeratoma
  Glomangioma
  Adenoma sebaceum
Melanocytic conditions
  Granuloma faciale
  Melanocytic nevus
  Nevus of Ota (dermal melanocytosis)
  Benign lentigo
  Lentigo maligna
  Chloasma (melasma)
  Cafe au lait spot
  Traumatic black tattoos
  Pigmented seborrheic keratoses
  Decorative black (red) tattoos

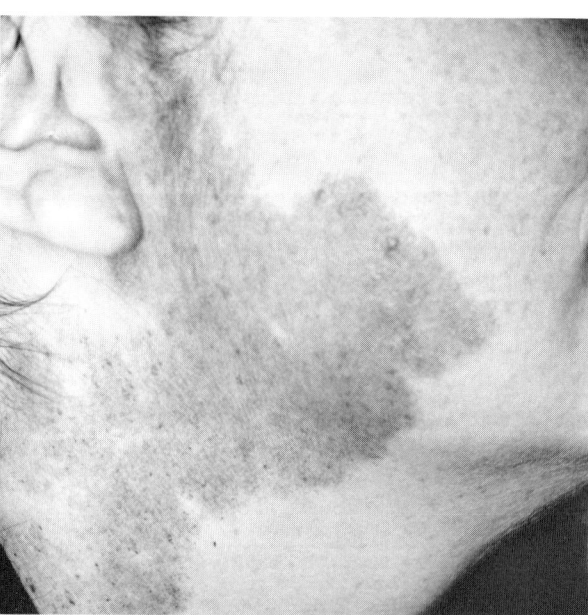

Figure 9. Preoperative appearance of an extensive angioma of the jaw and lateral neck.

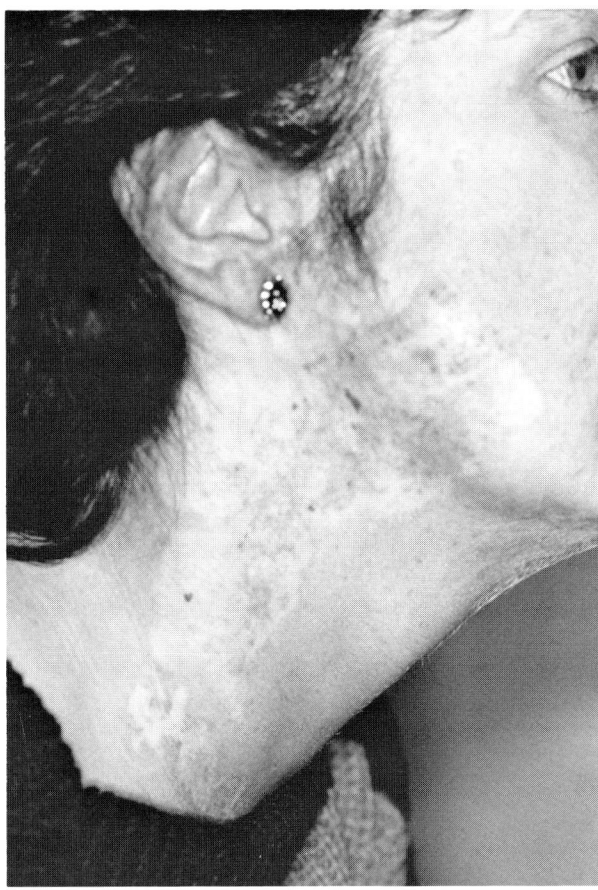

Figure 10. Appearance of the same patient in Figure 9 demonstrating almost complete resolution of angioma with slight hypopigmentation remaining.

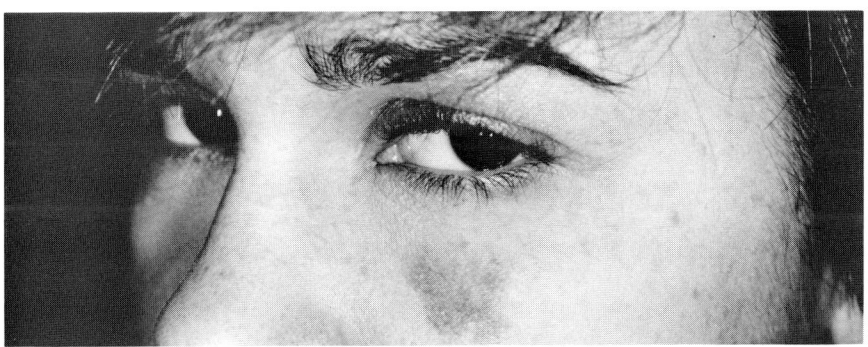

Figure 11. Small angioma of left upper cheek preoperatively.

Figure 12. The same patient as in Figure 11 showing almost complete resolution of angioma following argon laser photocoagulation therapy.

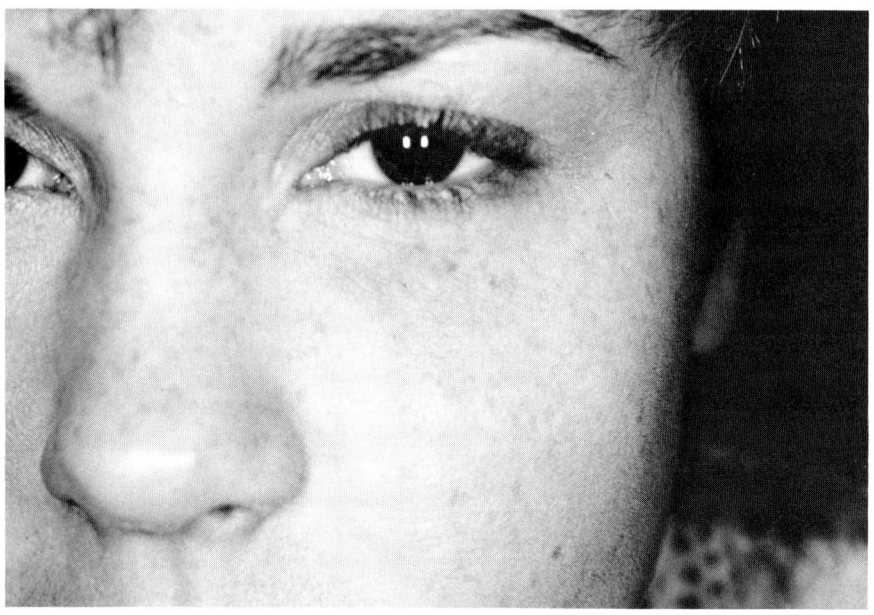

Figure 13. Preoperative clinical appearance of an extensive mid-facial angioma.

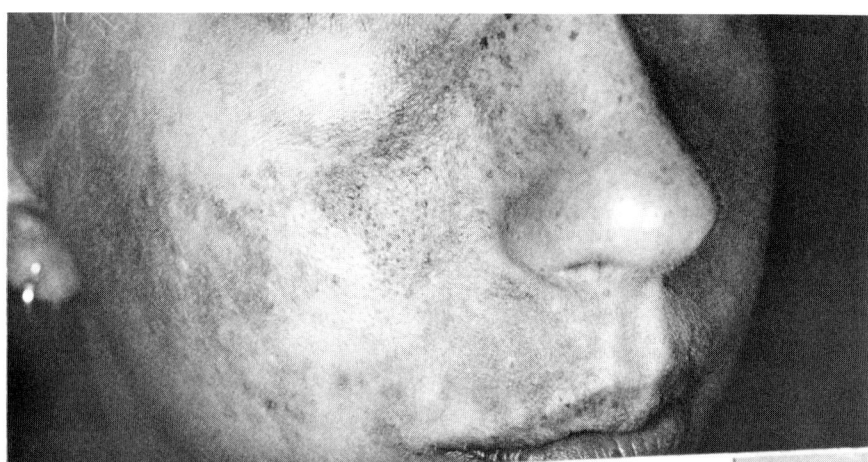

Figure 14. Appearance of same patient as in Figure 13 showing partial resolution of angioma but persistence of some vascular elements.

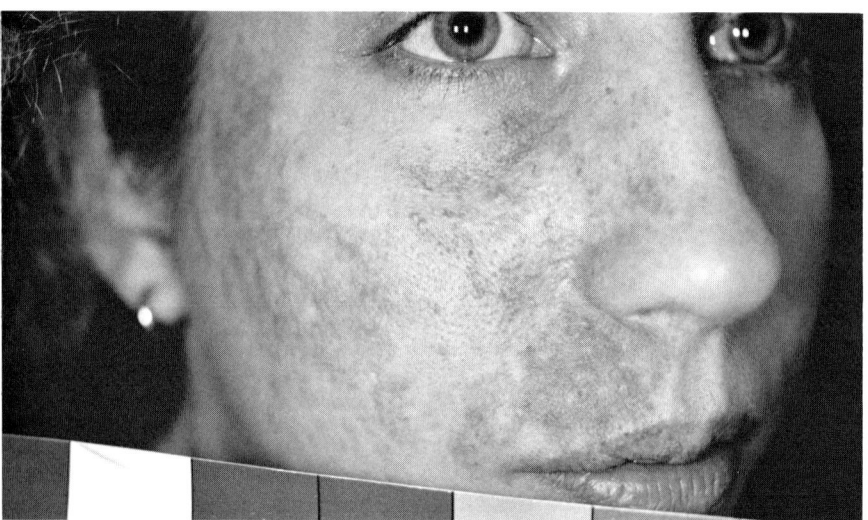

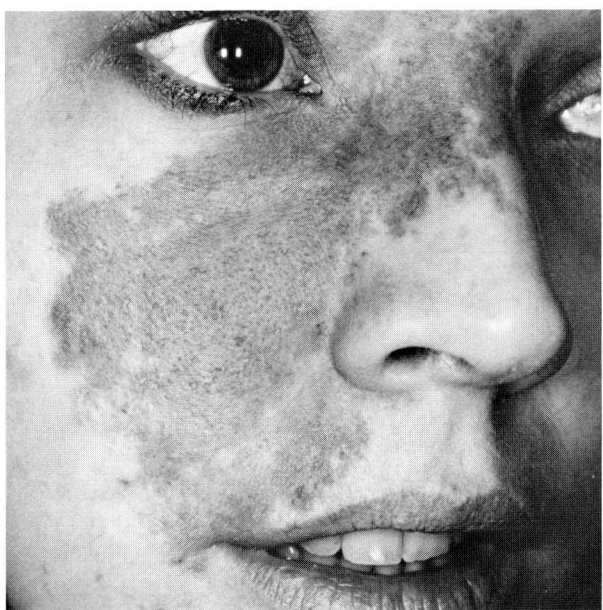

Figure 15. Preoperative appearance of midfacial angioma.

location. But, a patient with a deep red or blue-colored angioma would expect to see a proportionally greater improvement in color than a patient who presents with a light pink angioma. This is due to the fact that if the laser surgeon is able to reduce the amount of red or blue color of a deeply pigmented angioma by 70% to 80%, it may only be pink in color at the completion of laser therapy. However, 70% less pink color in a preexisting pink angioma is still likely to be pink and thus, the degree or quality of improvement may be only minimal in those cases. While these statistics are impressive, there are some unfortunate patients who show no lightening even many months after treatment and should not undergo further therapy.

While various lasers surgeons employ different techniques in the successful management of angiomas, there are some general principles that are employed by virtually all surgeons. The first area of controversy is the appropriate time at which to begin laser treatment for these lesions. It has been

Figure 16. Same patient as in Figure 15 demonstrating some persistent red color following argon laser treatment of the cheek and demonstrating that the mustache portion of the upper lip is frequently left untreated due to the risk of hypertrophic scarring.

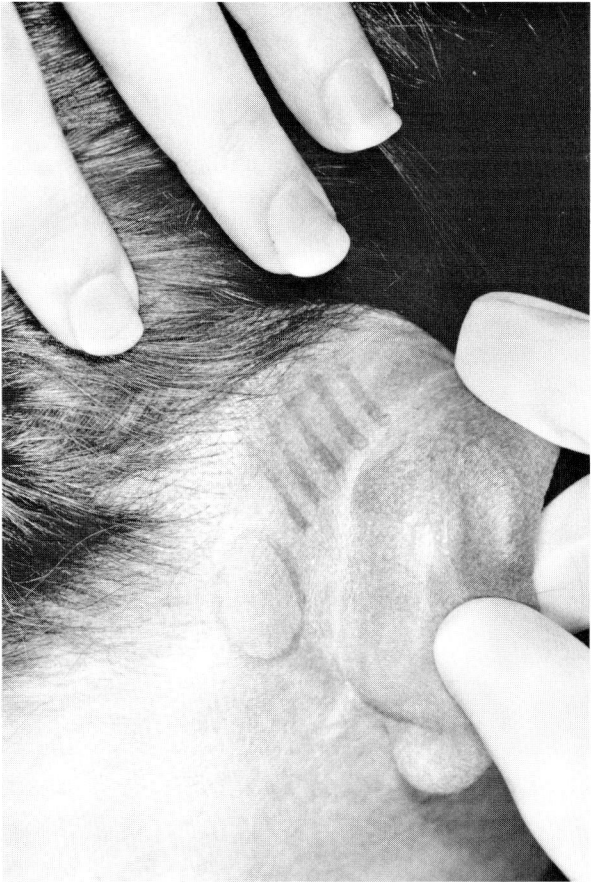

Figure 17. Retroauricular fold showing the planned test sites for both argon and carbon dioxide laser.

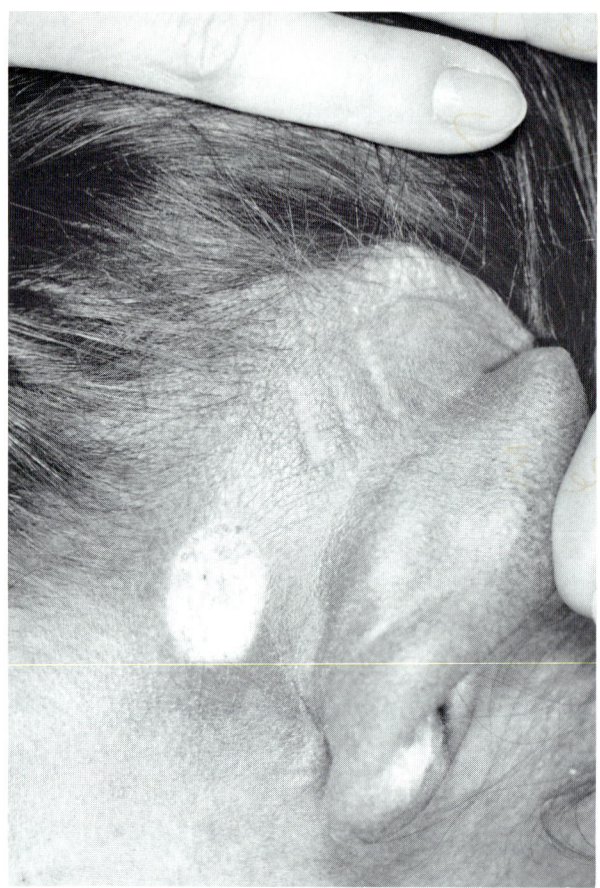

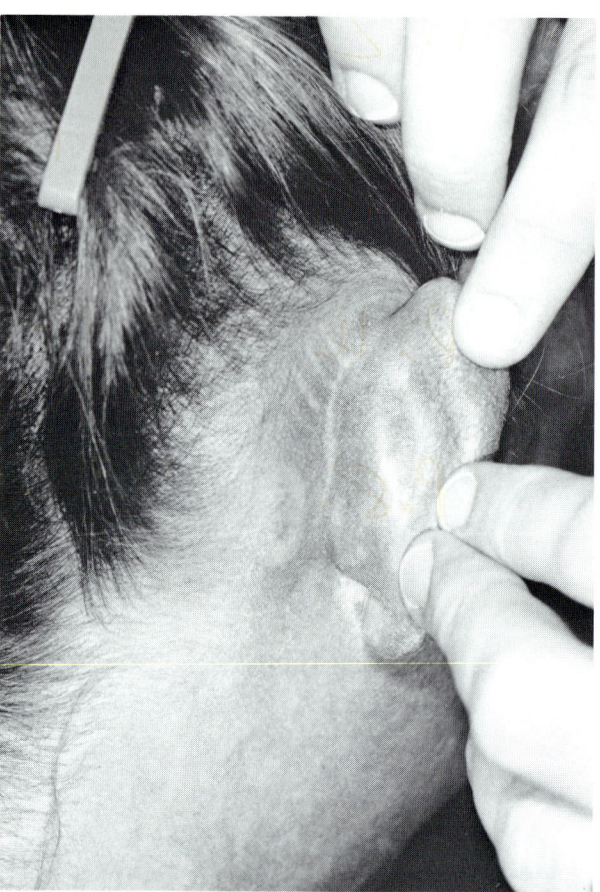

Figure 18. Appearance of same patient as in Figure 17 immediately after testing. The CO_2 test site is the most inferior and appears white since the char has been removed with hydrogen peroxide. There is only slight change noted at the argon test site which is artefactual due to protein coagulation.

Figure 19. Same patient as in Figure 17, three months postoperatively, showing early lightening of four of the argon test sites and some lightening of the carbon dioxide laser test site.

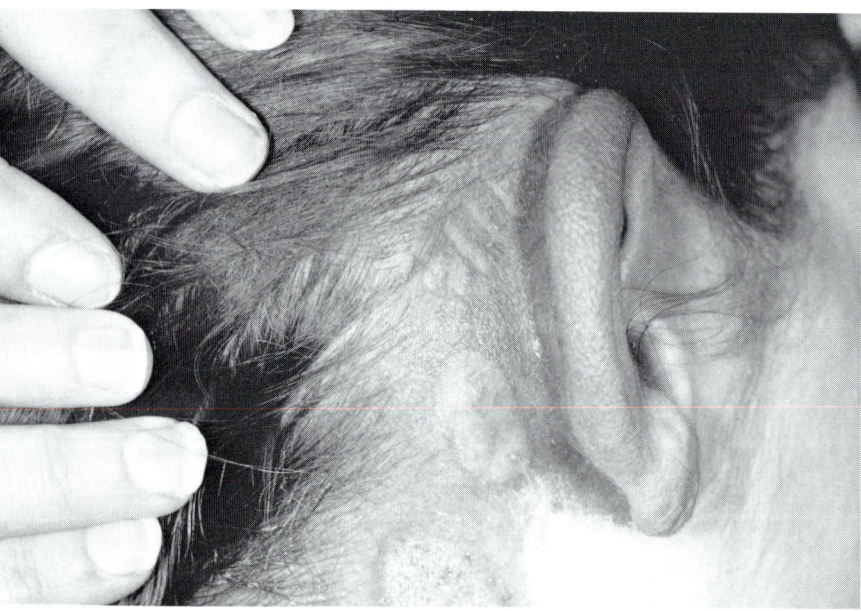

Figure 20. Same patient as in Figure 17, six months postoperatively, showing additional lightening with excellent texture at the argon test sites and lightening, but with some scarring at the CO_2 laser test site.

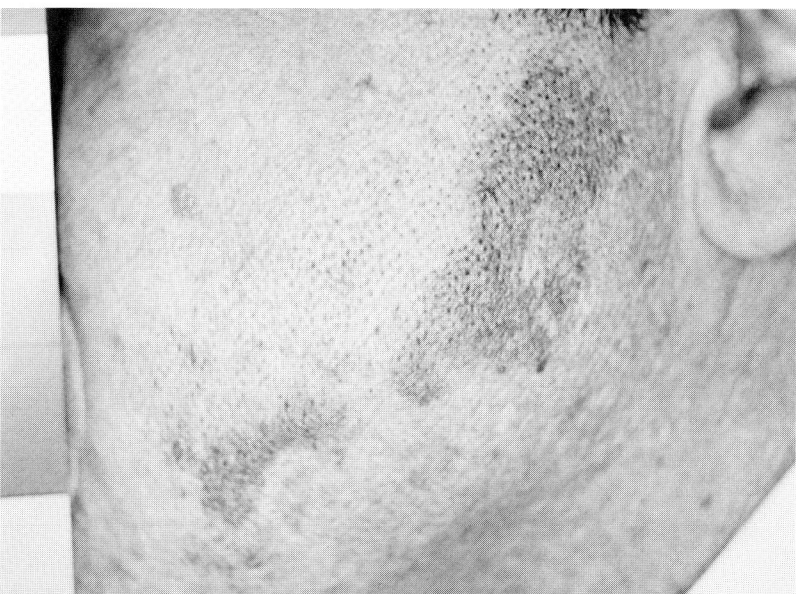

Figure 21. Preoperative appearance of a localized linear angioma of the left cheek.

known for some time that when surgical procedures are performed in children, the final cosmetic result obtained is usually less satifactory than if the procedure is performed as an adolescent or adult. This probably relates to the growth of the child and subsequent stretch of elastic tissues of the skin and mucous membranes. As a consequence, many laser surgeons do not offer the angioma patient any laser treatment until after puberty. However, recent results have indicated that with proper postoperative wound management, even young children 4 to 6 years of age can be successfully treated without complication using the argon laser.

Most laser surgeons will perform a test treatment to a representative portion of a portwine stain prior to beginning actual therapy. This test site is usually chosen in an inconspicuous area. This is commonly the postauricular area (Figures 17–20) (see color insert), or an area adjacent to the hairline (Figures 21–24) where if scarring or textural changes occur, they can generally be hidden by a minor change in hair style or by the surrounding normal anatomy. The test site itself is composed of four to six indiviual tests each representing a different combination of time, beam diameter, and irradiance (Figures 17 and 22). The immediate improvement which is manifest as blanching (Figures 18 and 23) does not accurately represent the final degree of improvement that can be seen. In fact, this immediate blanching represents protein coagulation of the epidermis and not a true representation of vascular effect at all. Consequently, even though the

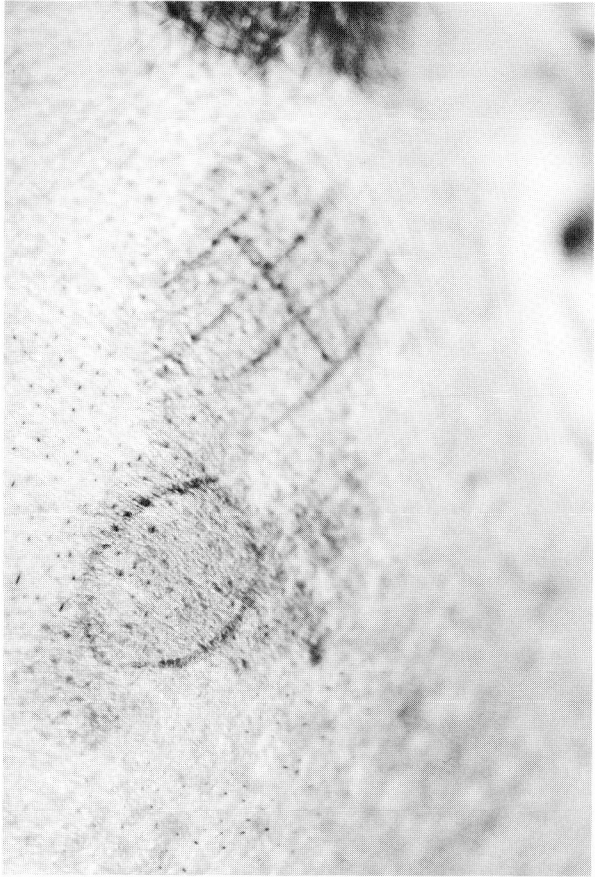

Figure 22. Appearance of the grid being established for argon and carbon dioxide laser testing.

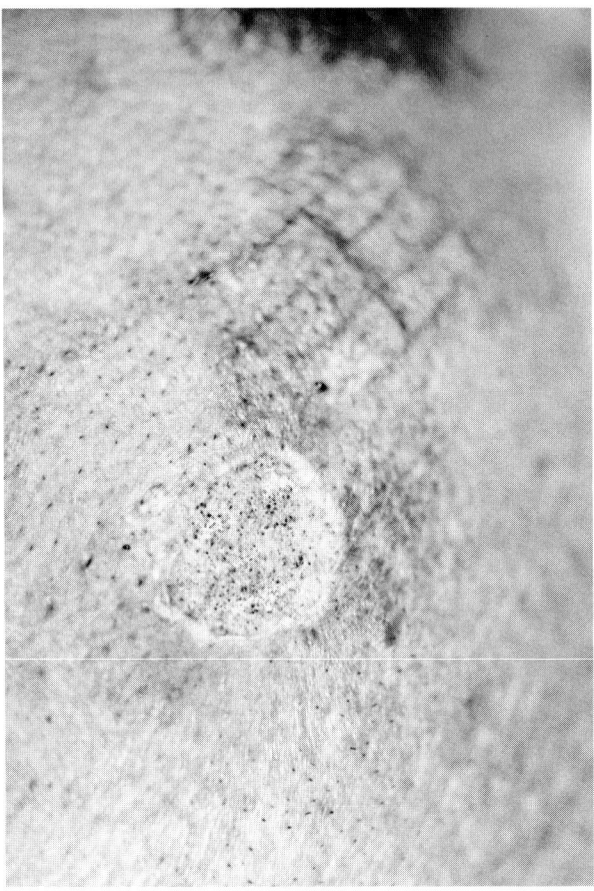

Figure 23. Appearance of test sites immediately after treatment. Slight blanching occurred at three argon test sites from protein coagulation. Superficial erosion with some crusting is seen at the circular carbon dioxide laser test site.

immediate results obtained with argon laser testing are recorded in the patient's record, they frequently do not correspond well with the final appearance that is seen three to six months later. Each small individual test is generally on the order of 2 to 3 mm in width by 8 to 10 mm in length. Local anesthesia may be employed as long as epinephrine is not utilized since this agent causes vasoconstriction and would decrease the volume of the hemoglobin target and possibly be responsible for less than optimal improvement.

Immediately after the test site has been treated, the wound is dressed with an antibacterial ointment and a small Band-aid dressing. The patient is instructed to expect epidermal blistering and, perhaps, a superficial erosion to develop as a consequence of thermal injury to the skin usually by the third day postoperatively. Wound care consists of twice daily cleansing with 3% hydrogen peroxide followed by application of an antibacterial ointment. This care is continued until the skin has completely reepithelialized, usually ten to 14 days. The patient should be warned in advance that there may not be substantial lightening immediately after the treatment site has healed. The permanent blanching of the angioma is not expected to occur for a minimum of three months and may, on occasion, require 12 months until the dermal vascular structures have been completely sealed off and removed.

Generally, the patient is reevaluated three months after argon laser phototesting (see Figures 19 and 24). If no improvement has oc-

Figure 24. Same patient as in Figure 22, three months after laser testing, showing an excellent response at the carbon dioxide laser test site with substantial lightening and excellent texture. A lesser degree of improvement in color is seen at the argon laser test area.

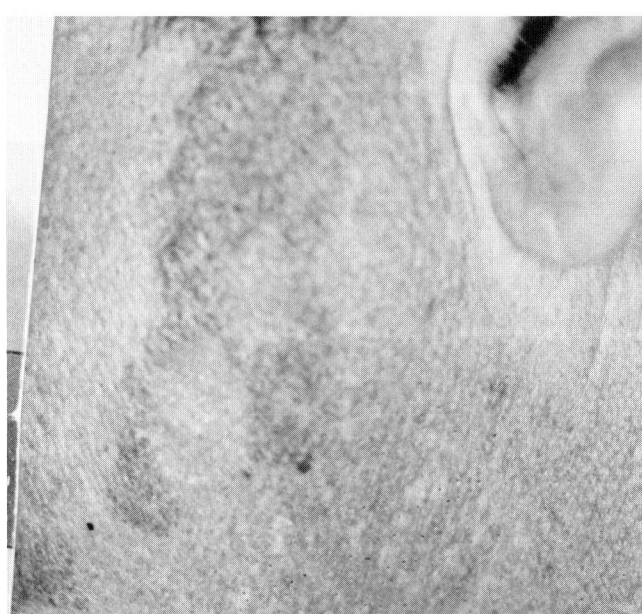

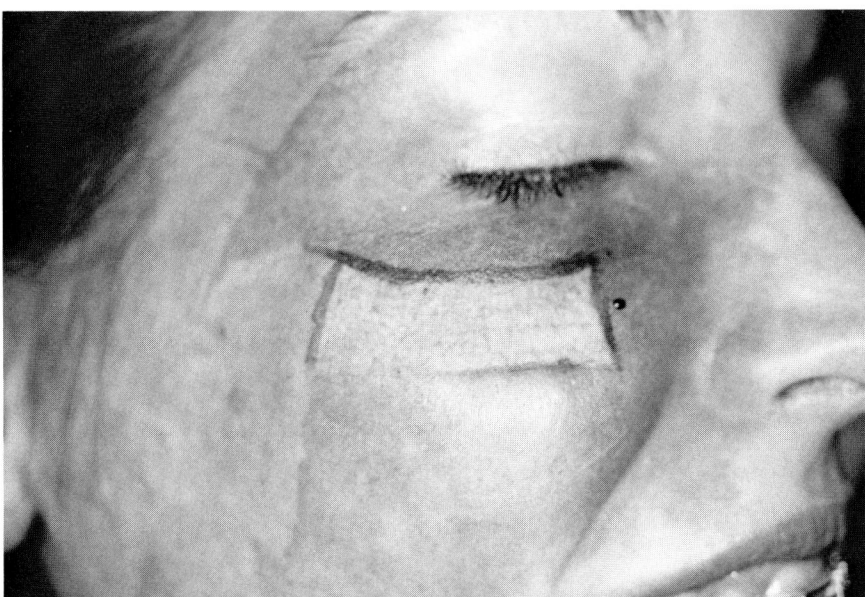

Figure 25. Clinical appearance of a standard treatment area for argon laser therapy of an angioma.

curred, treatment is delayed for an additional three months (Figure 20). At that time, the test sites are carefully examined and the quality of healing as well as the degree of lightening are both determined. If textural changes or adverse scarring, typically in the form of hypertrophic scars, have occurred, then additional treatment is contraindicated. If no textural change or scarring is noted and the degree of improvement has been substantial and the patient wishes to begin therapy, this may be initiated at that time.

The size of the individual treatment site is another point of some controversy among laser surgeons. Some feel that a zone of approximately 2 to 3 square inches (Figure 25) is all that should be treated at one time so the patient will be able to hide the treatment site relatively easily and not be cosmetically impaired during reepithelializa-

tion. Other laser surgeons will treat a substantial percentage of the angioma at each visit so that the treatment can be completed within six months from the time of onset. The major risk that occurs with this more aggressive form of therapy is related to possible secondary infection. A disastrous result may occur if a substantial portion of the face is treated and secondary infection occurs compromising the final cosmetic result. If the angioma is small, the entire lesion may be treated in one session (Figures 26–28). There is no one right answer as far as the size of the treatment size is concerned. If local anesthesia is required, it may limit the size of the treatment. The volume of the local anesthetic agent injected must be recorded to prevent any possible toxicity from occurring by use of excessive amounts of local anesthesia.

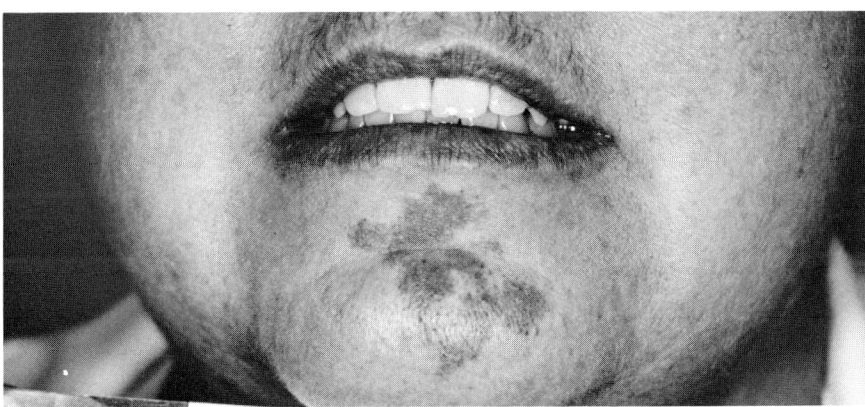

Figure 26. Preoperative appearance of an angioma of the chin.

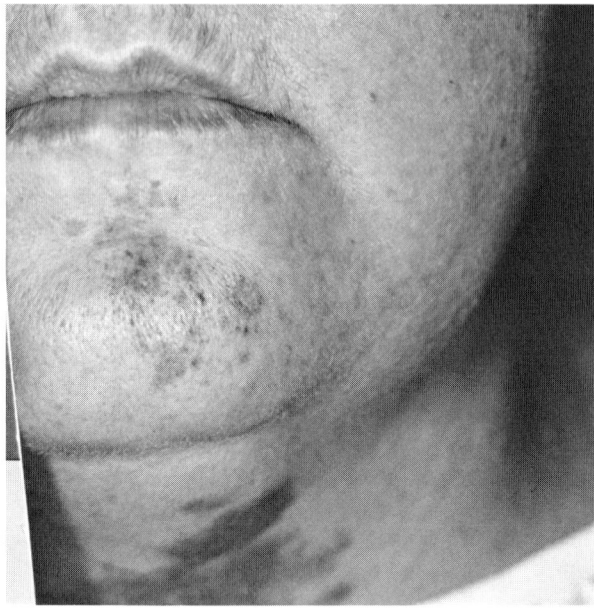

Figure 27. Appearance six weeks after argon laser photocoagulative therapy in patient shown in Figure 26.

can be tolerated without much difficulty by most patients. However, if the pulse duration required for improvement is .10 second in duration or longer, most individuals will not be able to tolerate this degree of heat for long. In those cases, either the size of the treatment area must be kept small or local anesthetic must be utilized.

The sensation the patient feels with a single laser pulse is one of very intense, but brief heat. It can be likened to the sensation that is associated with frying meats on a grill where small droplets of heated oil spatter into the air and briefly heats the skin. For the argon laser, while the sensation is intense, it is very brief and as long as some rest interval is permitted between pulses, the discomfort can be minimized. Virtually no patient is able to tolerate a continuous type of exposure to the argon laser beam because the discomfort is too great. In these cases, local anesthesia is obviously necessary. It should be remembered, however, that epinephrine is not added to the local anesthesia since this will cause vasconstriction and decrease the quantity of the red blood cell target which is required to absorb the argon laser energy.

Treatment sessions for large angiomas of the face are usually staggered at six-week intervals. This gives the individual sufficient time to heal completely before another treatment is performed. If possible, it is wise to deliver the laser

Some patients can tolerate the discomfort of argon laser therapy without difficulty. This is especially true if the optimal lightening has occurred after testing with pulse durations that are relatively short; then the amount of discomfort

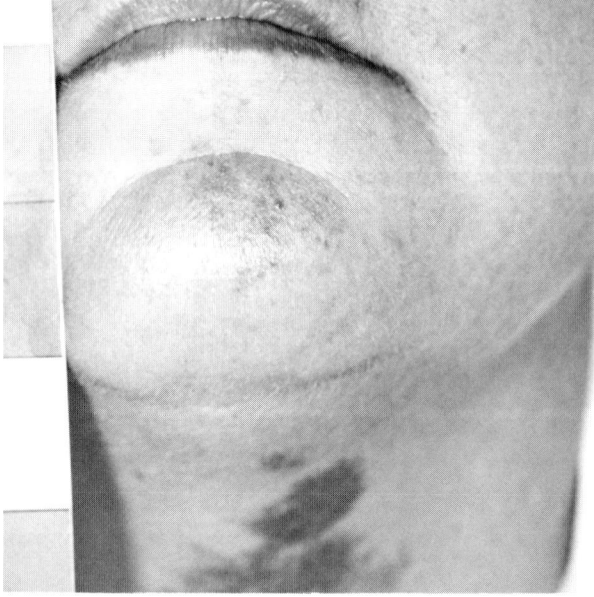

Figure 28. Appearance of same treatment site of patient in Figure 26, six months post-laser treatment, demonstrating almost complete resolution.

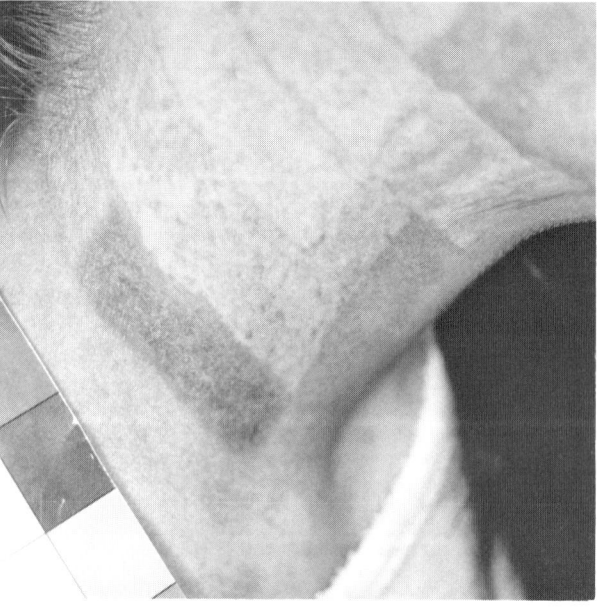

Figure 29. Postinflammatory hyperpigmentation of a test site of the right lateal neck following argon laser photocoagulation.

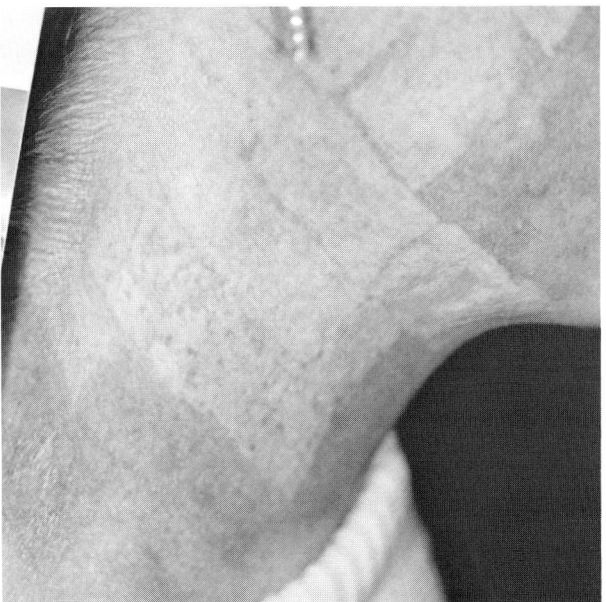

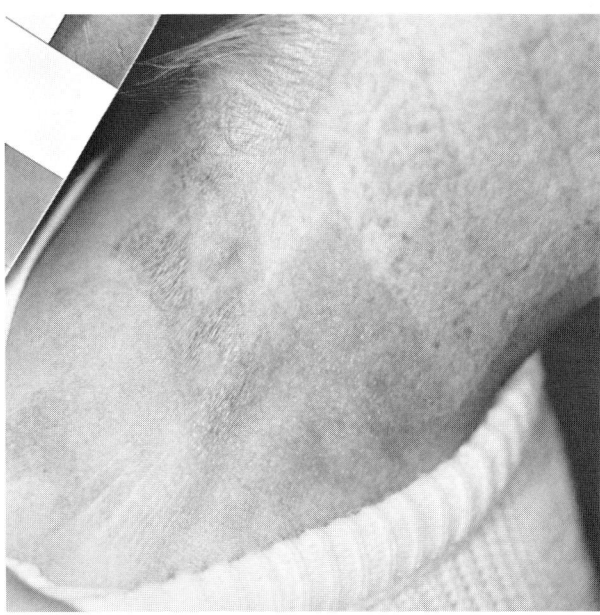

Figure 30. Jigsaw-puzzle type of appearance due to gradation of lightening from successive argon laser treatments.

Figure 31. Gradual blending in of the jigsaw-puzzle pattern as additional lightening occurs.

energy in the direction of natural skin creases, folds or relaxed skin tension lines to optimize the chances of a satisfactory cosmetic improvement. On a more practical level, there is a gradation in the degree of lightening seen when large angiomas are treated with the argon laser. In this way, the oldest treatment site is the lightest and the most recent treatment site remains the darkest in color since there is a slow but gradual diminution in color over a period of many months. This may result in a temporary jigsaw puzzle pattern as the various sections slowly lighten after treatment is completed (Figures 29–32).

If ice is applied to the treatment site immediately after laser treatment has been performed, there is usually less postoperative swelling and pain. For those individuals who are able to tolerate argon laser phototherapy without the need for local anesthesia, immediate application of ice will cool the heated tissue sufficiently to provide immediate relief. Wound care instructions are relatively simple as previously discussed. However, it is strongly recommended that the patient not expose treated areas directly to sunlight for a period of, at least, six months since postinflammatory hyperpigmentation may occur. While

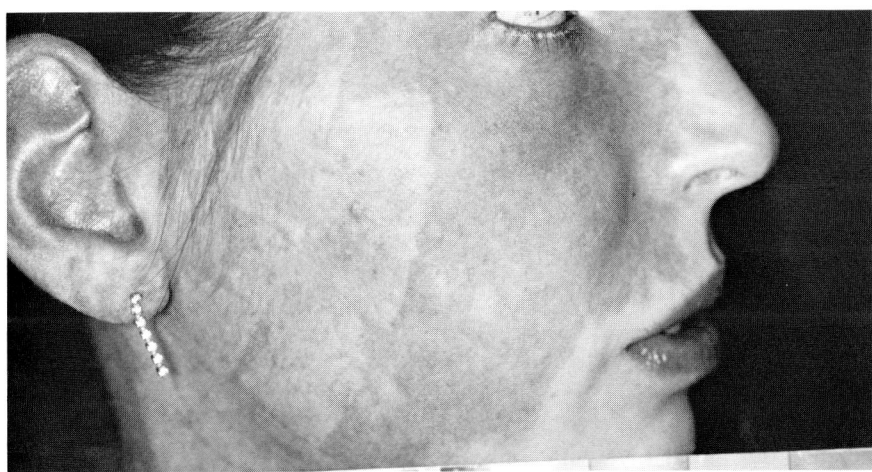

Figure 32. Same patient as demonstrated in Figure 29 showing similar jigsaw-pattern type of appearance with argon laser segmental treatment.

Figure 33. Severe hypertrophic scarring with distortion of the lip following argon laser treatment.

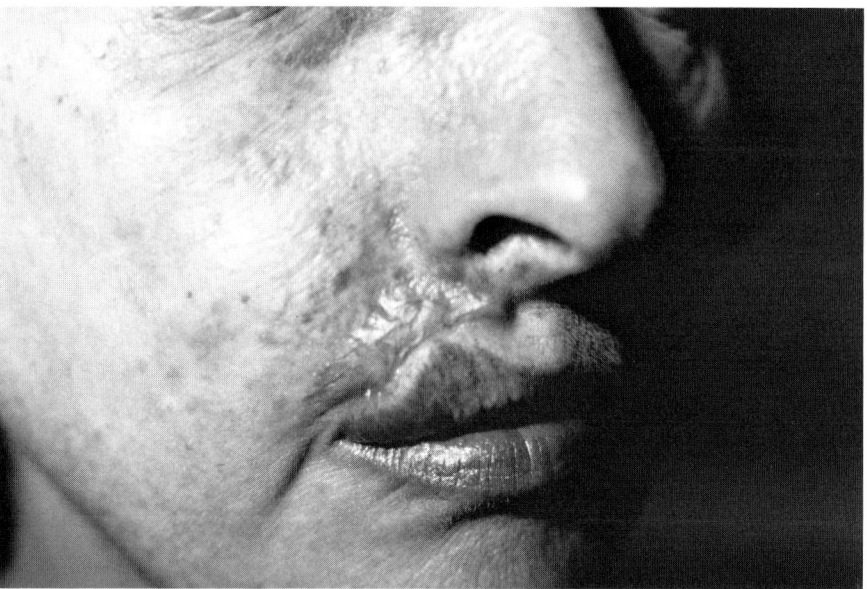

this color will eventually disappear with time, the cosmetic results may be impaired due to the brown discoloration which has replaced the original color of the angioma.

A period of at least 12 months should be given for lightening to occur prior to considering any retreatment. This is a function of the fact that lightening of angiomas following argon laser photocoagulation can continue for up to 18 months even though the greatest degree of improvement occurs in the first year postoperatively. If sufficient red color remains in the angioma after this interval, retreatment can be considered. However, in most cases, the degree of additional improvement that occurs with retreatment will not equal that seen with the first series of treatments. However, the additional improvement may be sufficient to warrant treatment in those individuals who are dissatisfied with the degree of improvement obtained after completion of the initial series of treatments.

There are special considerations that must be observed when performing argon laser treatment in several anatomic sites. The first of these is on the mustache portion of the upper lip. For reasons that are not entirely clear, this anatomic site is highly subject to hypertrophic scarring (Figure 33). If the same parameters are used on the upper lip as were employed for treatment of the remainder of the angioma on the face, hypertrophic scarring may occur in spite of the fact that the remainder of the treated sites have healed without difficulty. As a consequence, a different technique is utilized in the treatment of the

upper lip with small areas treated at each session creating a checkerboard-type pattern (Figures 34–37). This polka dot process is continued at six-week intervals until the entire lip has been treated with slightly overlapping dots of argon laser energy (Figures 38–41). This technique now permits successful treatment of the upper lip with the same degree of improvement obtained on the remainder of the face (Figures 42 and 43).

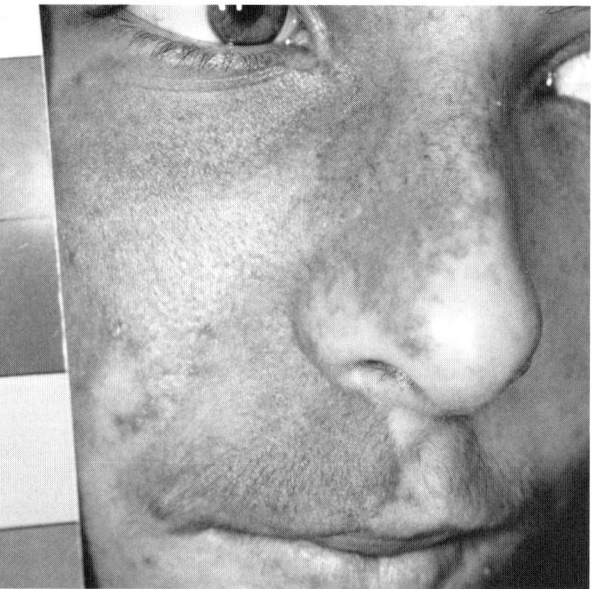

Figure 34. Preoperative appearance of the angioma of the central face and upper lip.

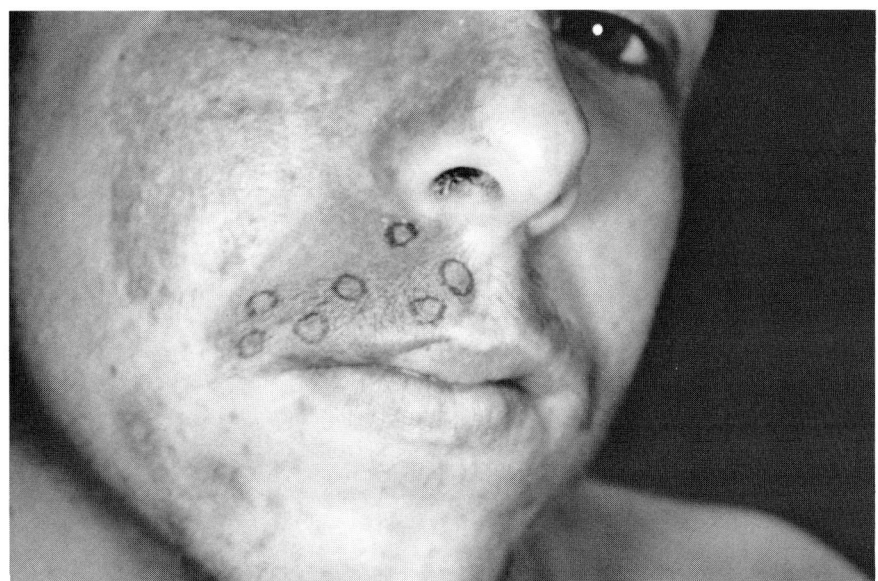

Figure 35. Same patient as in Figure 34 with small 2 to 3 mm circular areas outlined with a surgical marker prior to argon laser treatment.

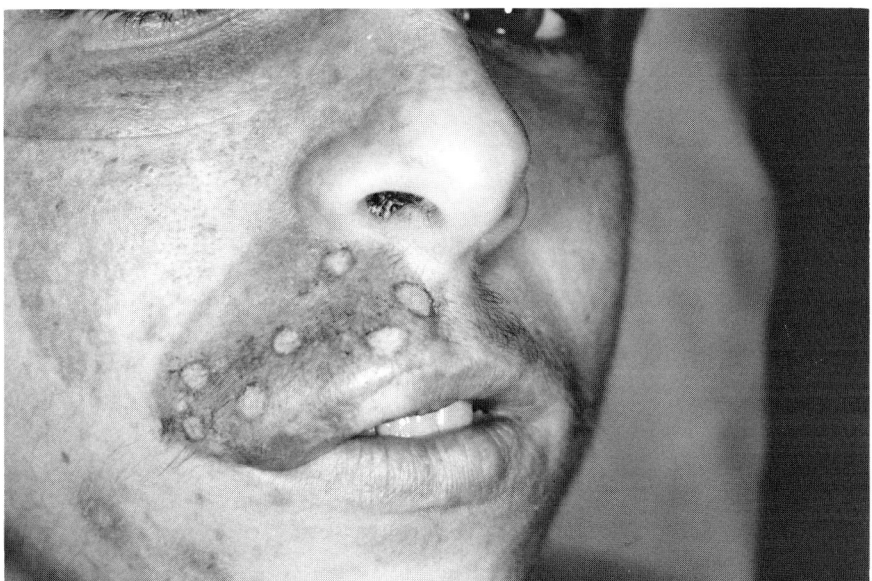

Figure 36. Same patient as in Figure 34 immediately after argon laser photocoagulative therapy to grid-like pattern of lip.

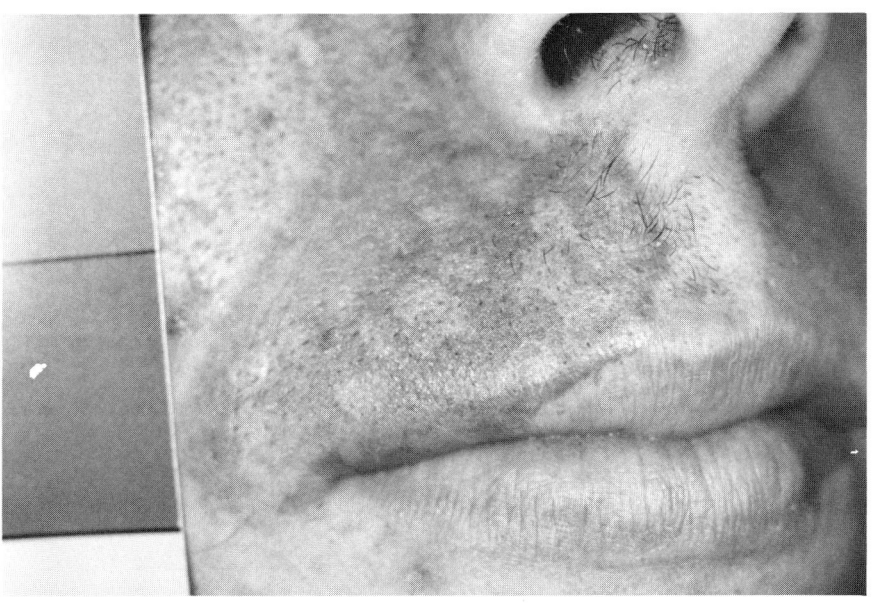

Figure 37. Lightening of the areas treated on the upper lip outlined in Figure 35, six weeks postoperatively.

Figure 38. Clinical appearance preoperatively of a small angioma of the upper lip.

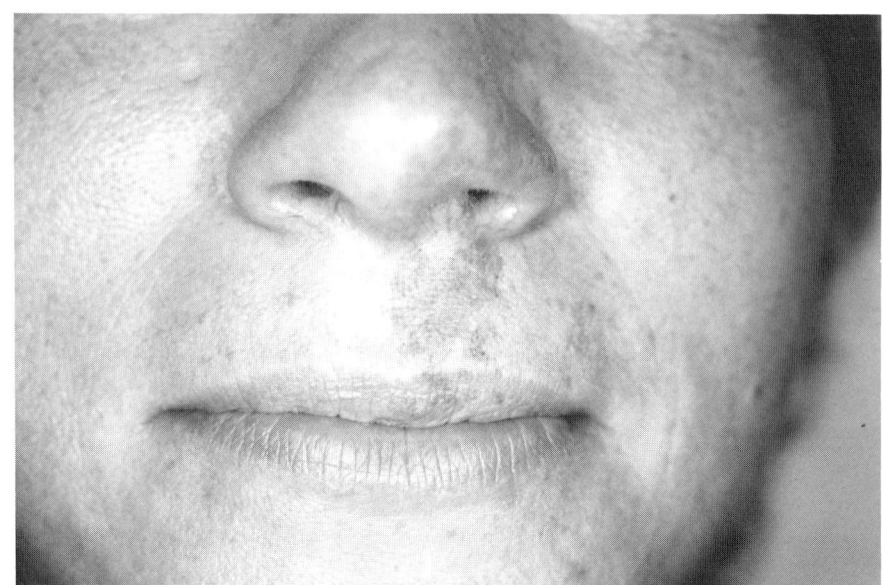

Figure 39. Appearance immediately after argon laser phototherapy showing superficial blanching at the points of energy delivery which represents protein coagulation and not true vascular effect.

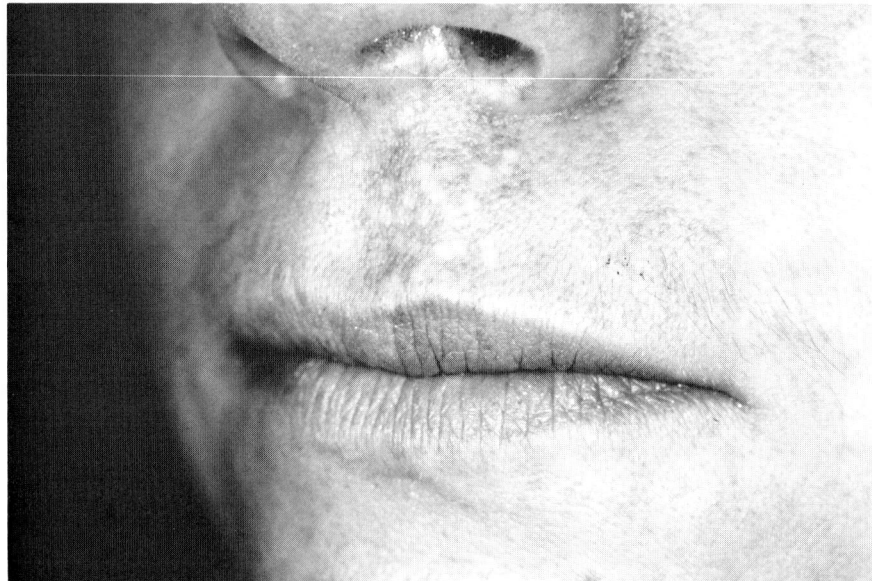

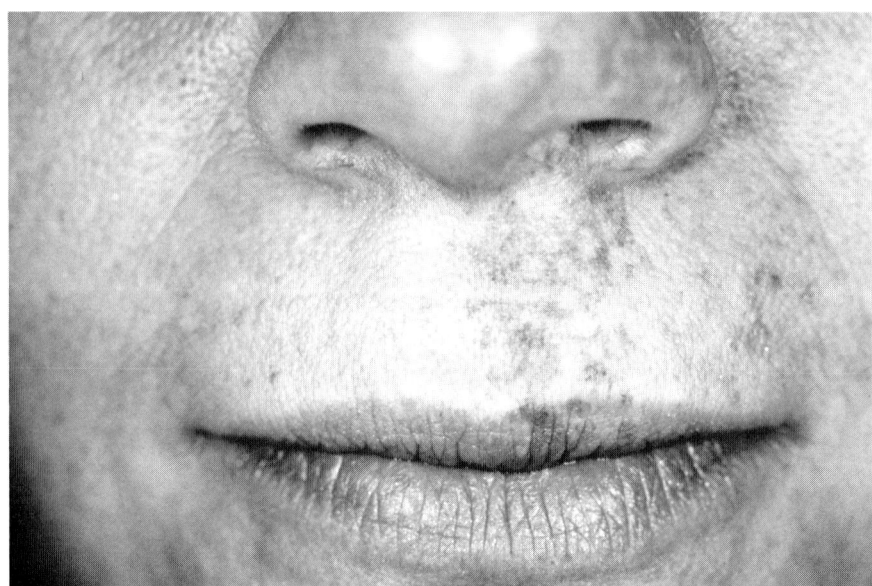

Figure 40. Appearance six weeks after treatment; permanent lightening and grid-like pattern can still be seen.

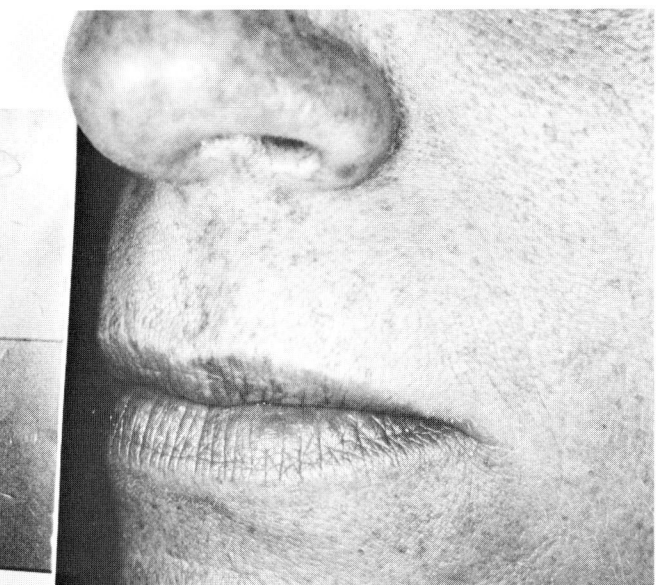

Figure 41. Appearance six months after treatment showing almost complete resolution of angioma of the upper lip without scarring or textural change.

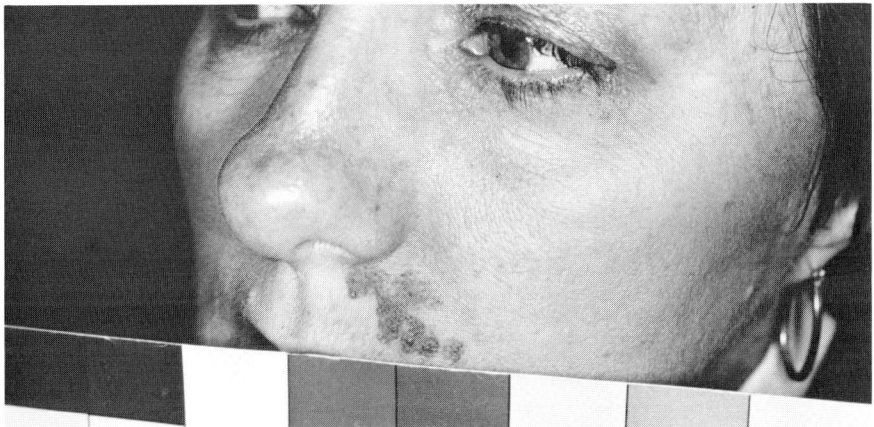

Figure 42. Preoperative appearance of a small angioma of the upper lip.

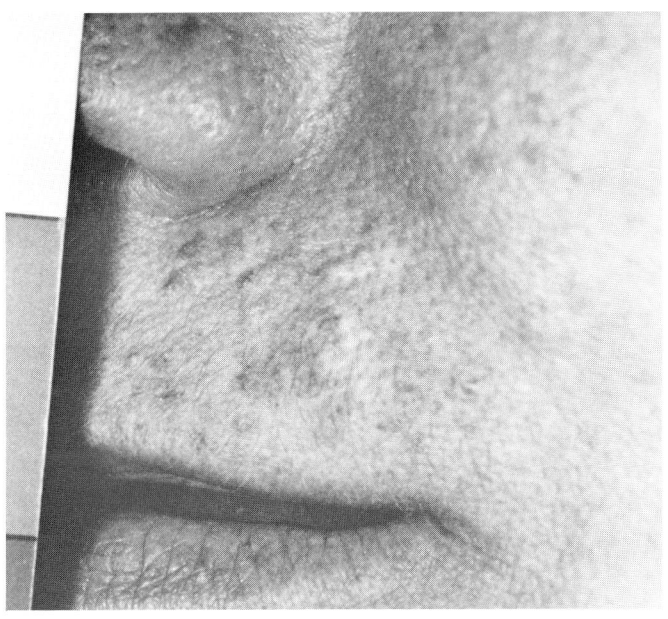

Figure 43. Almost complete resolution after argon laser treatment has been delivered in a grid-like pattern.

Figure 44. Cotton gauzes and plastic goggles are placed over the patient's eyes while working on the midcheek away from the orbit.

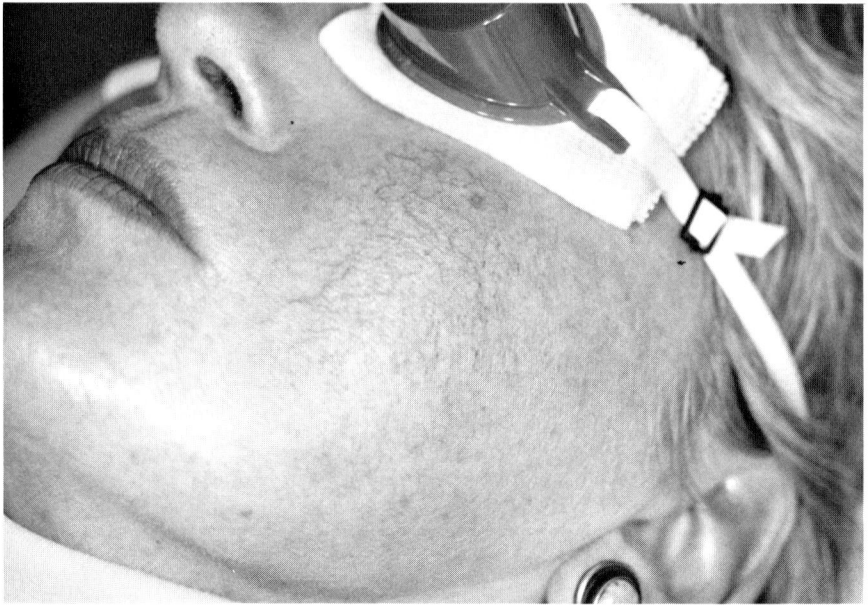

The second anatomic site that is of particular concern with argon laser photocoagulation therapy is the periorbital area. If the angioma involves both upper and lower lids as well as the ciliary margin, laser treatment can be safely performed as long as the eye is protected from inadvertent injury by the argon laser beam. If the laser surgeon is not working directly on the eyelids, a simple pair of plastic goggles placed over the eyes (Figure 44) will protect them completely. However, if the ciliary margin is being treated, safety precautions should include the application of a metal or plastic contact lens eyeshield (Figures 45–47) on the corneal surface prior to institution of argon laser therapy. These devices, which come in a variety of different styles and sizes, permit the safe treatment of angiomas even extending onto the ciliary margin. Topical anes-

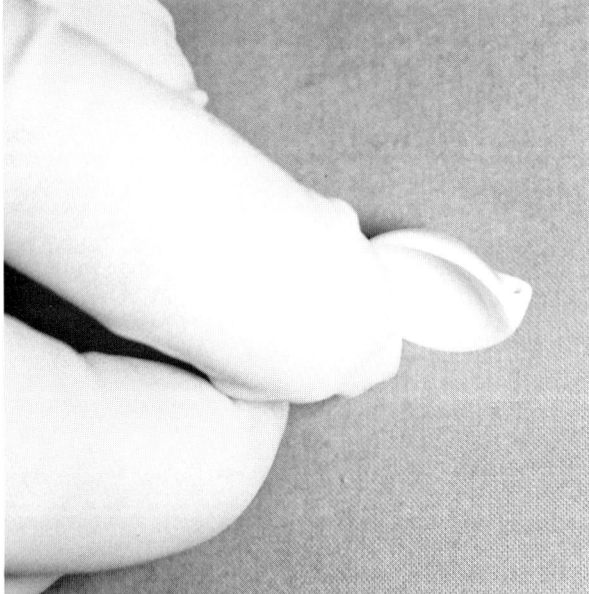

Figure 45. Concave surface of Hornblass ocular protective shield.

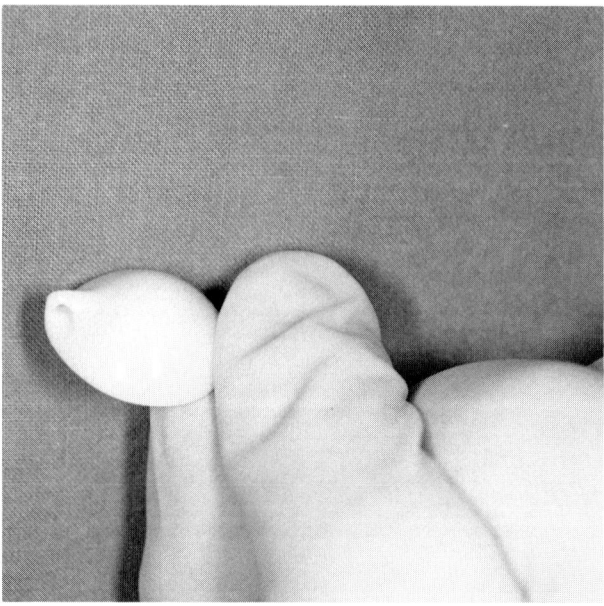

Figure 46. Convex surface of Hornblass ocular protective shield showing fenestrated handle for placement.

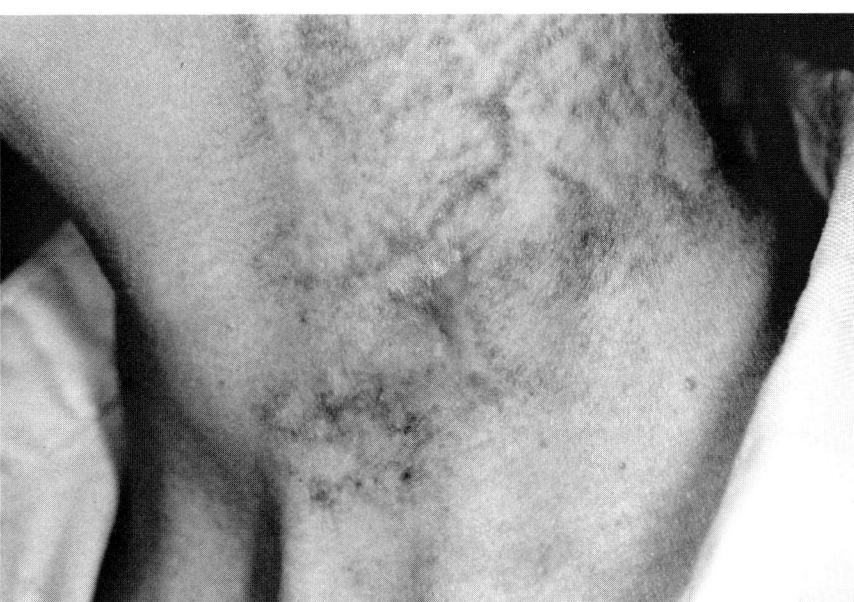

Figure 58. Weblike hyperpigmentation at various argon laser treatment sites of the lateral neck three months postoperatively.

neck and jawline. These very mobile portions of the facial anatomy are probably responsible for this type of scarring which occurs more readily than is seen with the less mobile portions of the face. Whether this is the main reason is not entirely clear, but each patient must be advised in advance about this possible outcome.

Another complication that is seen following argon laser therapy of angiomas is variation in pigmentation of the skin. Temporarily after treatment there may be slight hyperpigmenta-

tion (Figure 58), but this may be later replaced by hypopigmentation (Figure 59). This is due to absorption of argon laser energy by melanocytes, which causes their destruction in some patients, leading to permanent color changes at the treatment site.

Also to be avoided is the technique once commonly employed where linear stripes of laser energy were delivered to the surface of the angioma sparing small amounts of skin in between. Patients treated in this way (Figure 60) often ob-

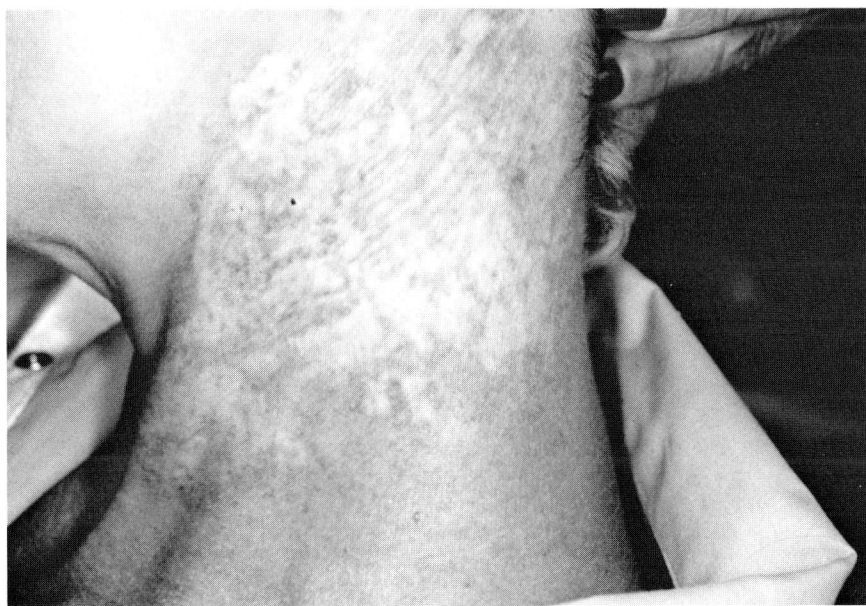

Figure 59. Hypopigmentation has now replaced areas of hyperpigmentation due to inadvertent damage to melanocytes of the skin by the argon laser.

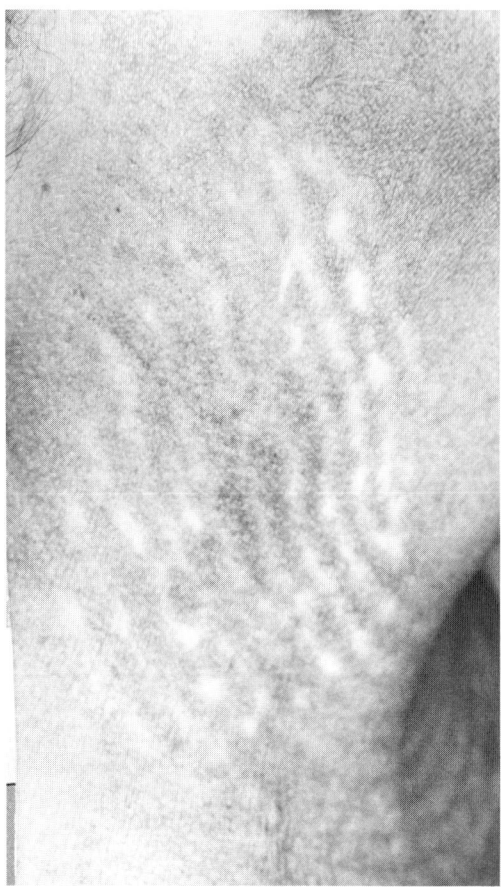

Figure 60. Striping technique previously used to treat angiomas showing prominent cosmetic disfigurement.

tained poor cosmetic results and much greater difficulty occurred when later attempting to blend in all the treatment sites.

ARGON LASER SAFETY

The argon laser used in the treatment of mucocutaneous disorders is classified as a type IV laser which is the designation for the most dangerous type of laser systems currently available. In order to utilize these instruments with the greatest degree of safety, several precautions must be taken. The first is a simple posting on the laser operating-room door that a laser is in use. The type of laser being employed should be identified so that glasses or goggles of proper optical density can be used before entering. Some laser operating suites have an interlock system that makes the operating room door impossible to open as long as the laser is in use. If the argon laser operating suite has an exterior window, the window must be covered to prevent inadvertent injury to observers outside the operating room. The visible blue-green argon laser light can pass through glass without difficulty and as a consequence, there is potential harm to outsiders.

The greatest risk for the argon laser is that of potential eye injury if the laser is inadvertently fired at the patient, surgeon, or assistant. When using the argon laser, if protection is not used, permanent injury to the retina can occur. If one remembers that this form of laser energy, ab-

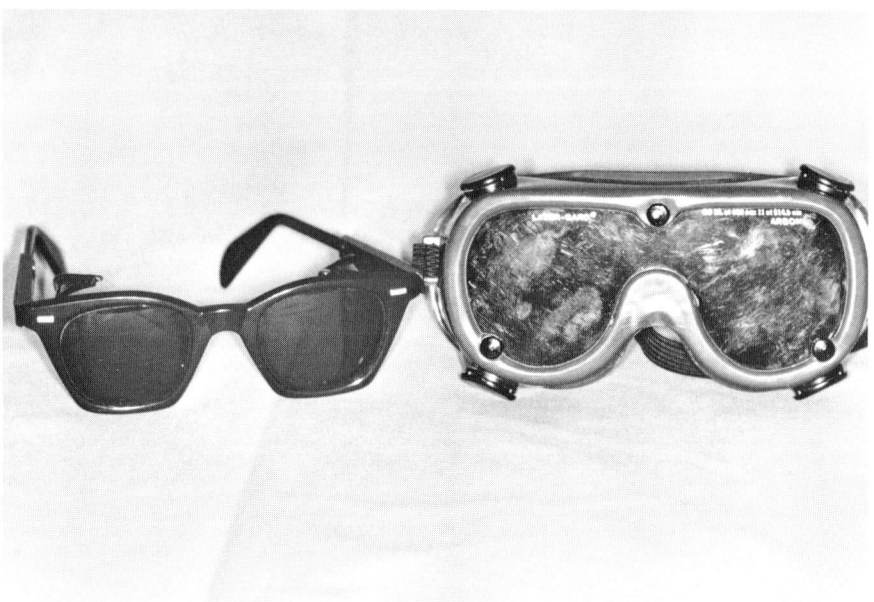

Figure 61. Various types of eye protection used with argon laser treatment.

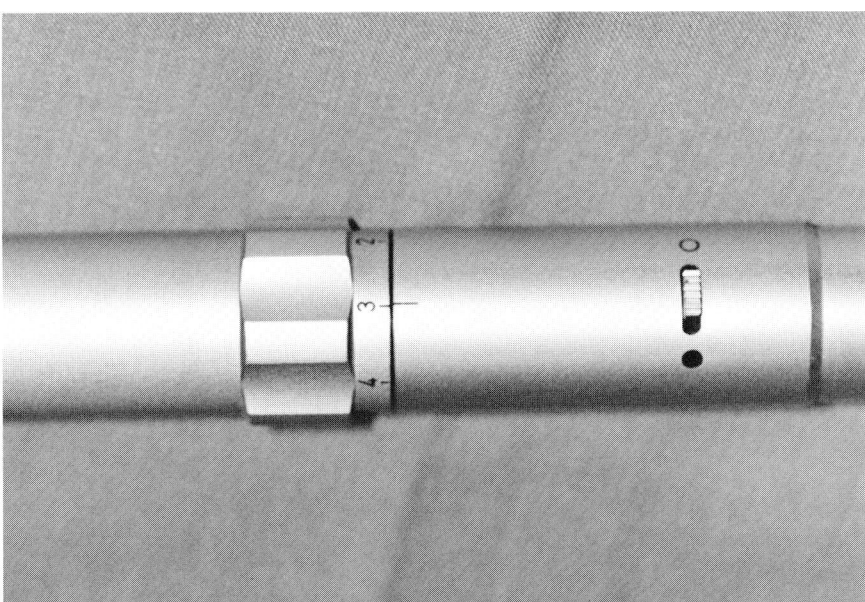

Figure 62. Close-up showing aperture on handpiece of argon laser which is kept in a closed position after the laser is activated to prevent inadvertent injury to the eyes.

sorbed by melanin and hemoglobin, has been utilized by ophthalmologists for years in the treatment of a variety of degenerative conditions of the retina, then it can be readily understood that inadvertent retinal damage can also occur resulting in permanent vision loss. For the visible light lasers, such as the argon laser, the laser energy can be focused by the patient's own lens on to the fovea of the eye. For this reason, eye protection is required by all operating room personnel as well as the patient whenever the argon laser is employed. For most individuals, this eye protection consists of simple plastic lenses or goggles of proper optical density (Figure 61) that can be worn over regular prescription lenses or in place of prescription lenses during argon laser surgery. The specific optical density of these plastic lenses absorbs the various wavelengths of light emitted by the argon laser from 488 nm to 514 nm. As previously discussed, when working directly upon the eyelids or the ciliary margin, eyeshields of either plastic or steel design are utilized to limit the risk of injury to the retina.

Three additional components are designed to further improve the safe operation of the argon laser. The first is an aperature on the laser hand-

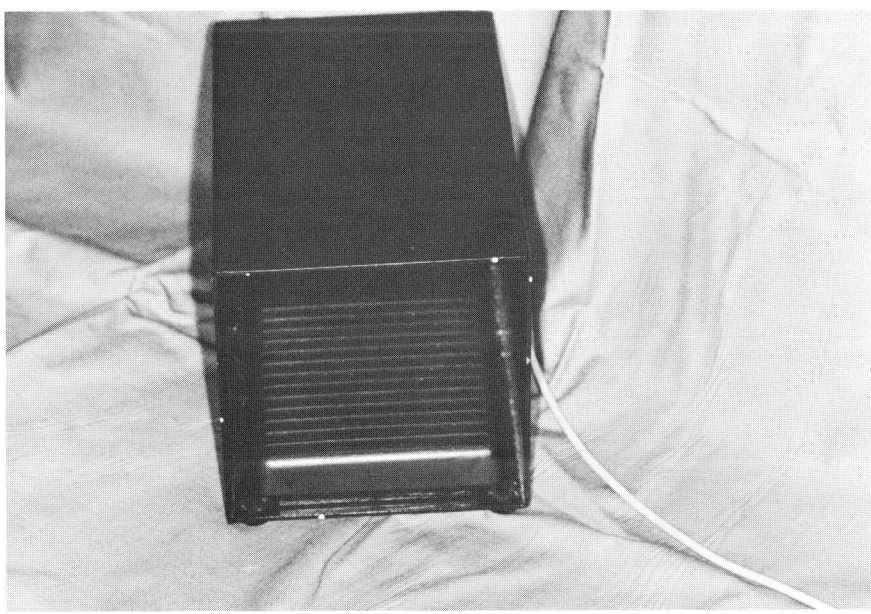

Figure 63. Box-like housing around argon laser foot pedal.

Figure 64. Emergency off-button is seen in the center of the argon laser control panel.

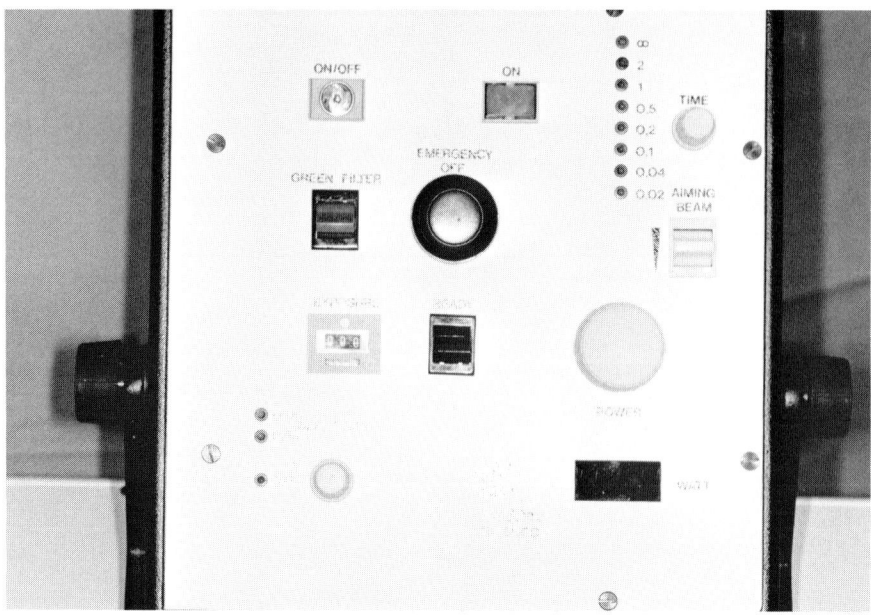

piece (Figure 62) which has an open and closed position. Each time the laser is first turned on, the aperature should be closed so no inadvertent discharge of laser energy can occur. The second is a box-like compartment that houses the laser foot pedal (Figure 63) to prevent accidental discharge of argon laser energy by a misplaced foot. Third, is an emergency off switch or panic button (Figure 64) found on the laser console which is used to shut the entire system down immediately if some problem occurs during treatment.

ARGON LASER PHOTOCOAGULATION OF TELANGIECTASIA

The argon laser has also been used extensively in the treatment of a variety of other vascular conditions. One of the most common of these is the simple telangiectasia. Telangiectasias may form at any age (Figures 65 and 66) as a side effect of certain medications, chronic sunlight exposure, pregnancy, aging, genetic conditions, and some primary diseases of the skin. They are commonly present on the central face and in the perialar groove as well as on the nose itself and may be single (Figures 67–69), mat-like (Figures 70 and 71) or diffuse (Figures 72 and 73) in nature. While always benign, the condition, nonetheless, may cause sufficient disfigurement so that many patients will present for treatment of them.

The primary treatment previously used for this condition was the insertion of a small platinum wire electric needle into or around the affected vessel, followed by delivery of a short pulse of electrical current. If the placement of the needle tip was sufficiently close to the vessel, thermal

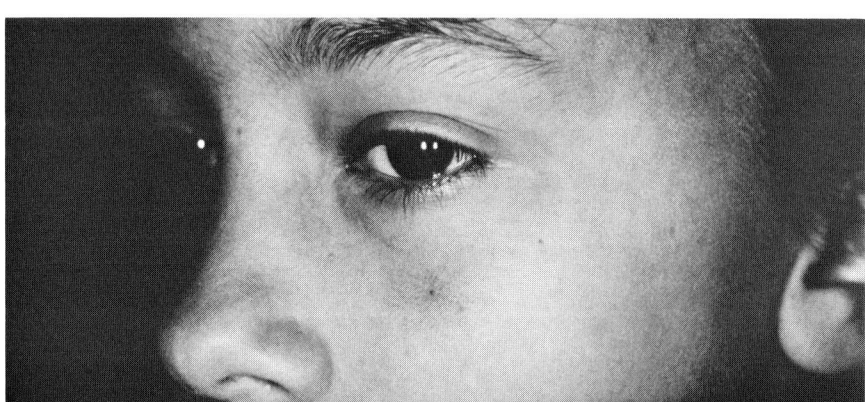

Figure 65. Small telangiectatic blood vessel of the midcheek in a young man.

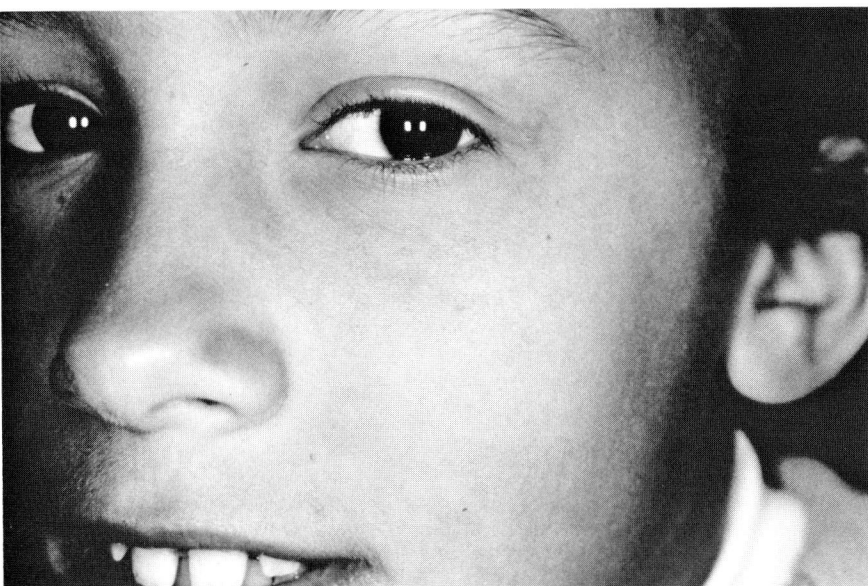

Figure 66. Same individual as in Figure 65 showing virtually complete resolution after argon laser treatment.

injury occurred and the vessel slowly resolved. Unfortunately, there was always some inadvertent thermal injury where the needle penetrated the intact skin, and occasionally resulted in a small pitted scar. As a consequence of this potential risk of scarring, as well as the commonly unsuccessful nature of this procedure, the argon laser has been substituted with great success in the management of this condition.

Since telangiectasias do not lend themselves well to testing with a number of different laser

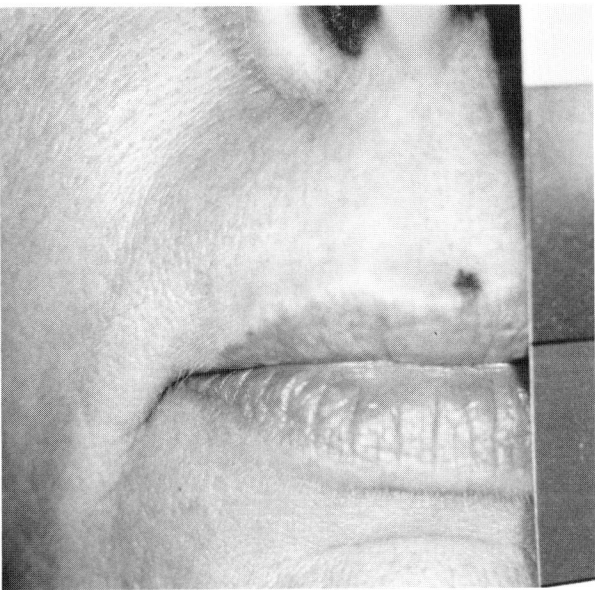

Figure 67. Single telangiectasia of the upper lip preoperatively.

parameters, in general, only one laser setting is utilized as a trial. Test sites are still recommended prior to initiating treatment of a large number of telangiectasias, even though the risk of adverse scarring or textural change with this treatment is relatively small. This small test is usually performed on an inconspicuous part of the face, such as the alar groove. Thus, if scarring should occur, it would not be noticeable in most cases.

Usually, within six weeks after testing, there has been substantial improvement. If adverse scarring has not occurred, then therapy can be initiated at that time. The effects of argon laser energy on telangiectasias is essentially identical to that described previously for the treatment of angiomas. The interaction between hemoglobin found within the dilated vessels and the blue-green argon laser energy results in transduction of the light energy into thermal energy which causes vascular injury, coagulation, and vessel resorption.

For this procedure, local anesthesia is not employed since it decreases the volume of blood present which, in turn, effectively decreases the size of the laser target and lessens the likelihood of a successful outcome. Standard parameters used in the treatment of telangiectasias are: a beam width of 0.5 mm, an energy setting of three watts, and a pulse duration of 0.04 seconds. This results in an irradiance of 1,530 watts/cm^2.

Using these settings, individual pulses are delivered along the length of each telangiectatic blood vessel until complete blanching occurs

Figure 68. Same patient as in Figure 67 showing improvement of color at four weeks post-laser treatment.

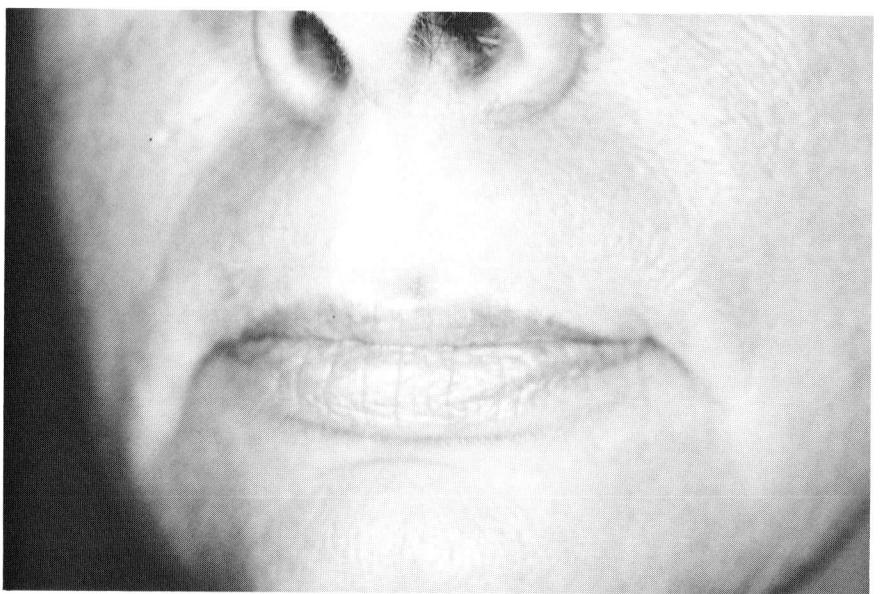

Figure 69. Same patient seen in Figure 67. Final appearance six months after treatment showing no persistent vascular structures and no clinical scarring or textural change.

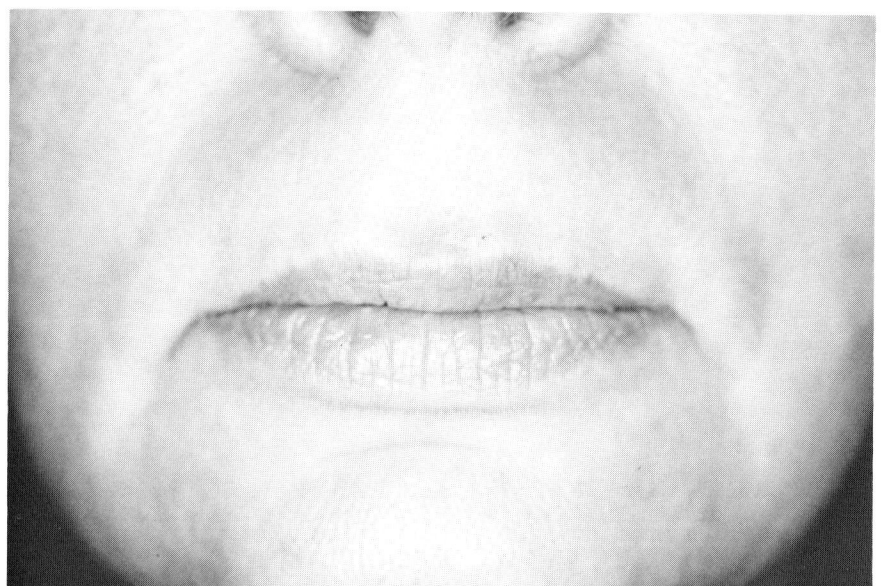

Figure 70. Mat-like collection of telangiectasias of the outer canthus.

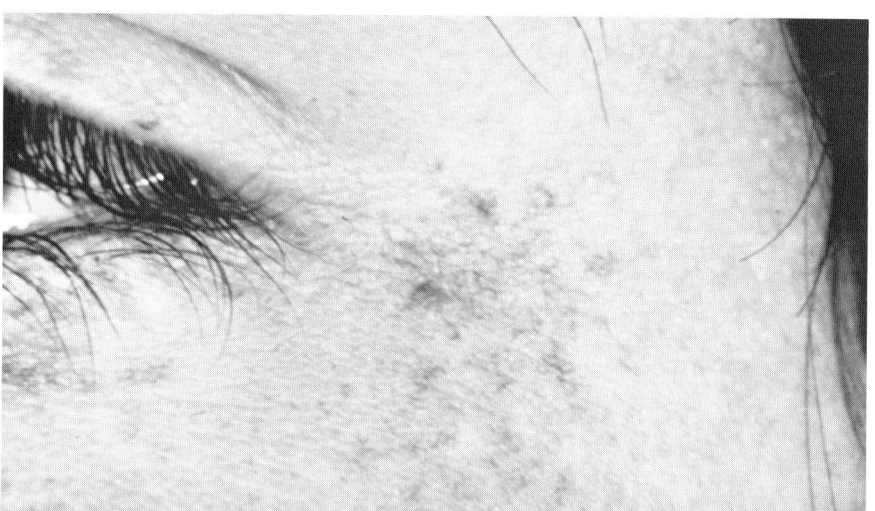

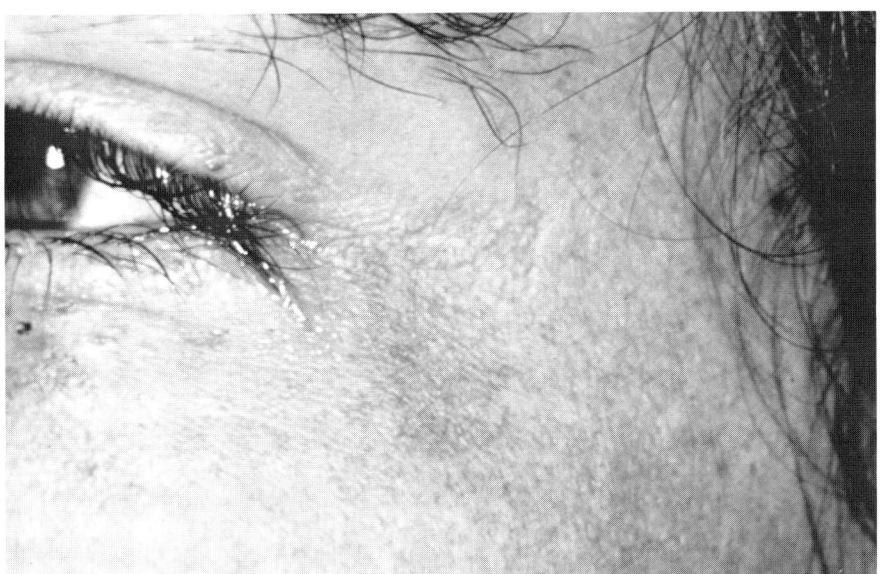

Figure 71. Same patient as in Figure 70 showing virtually complete resolution after argon laser treatment.

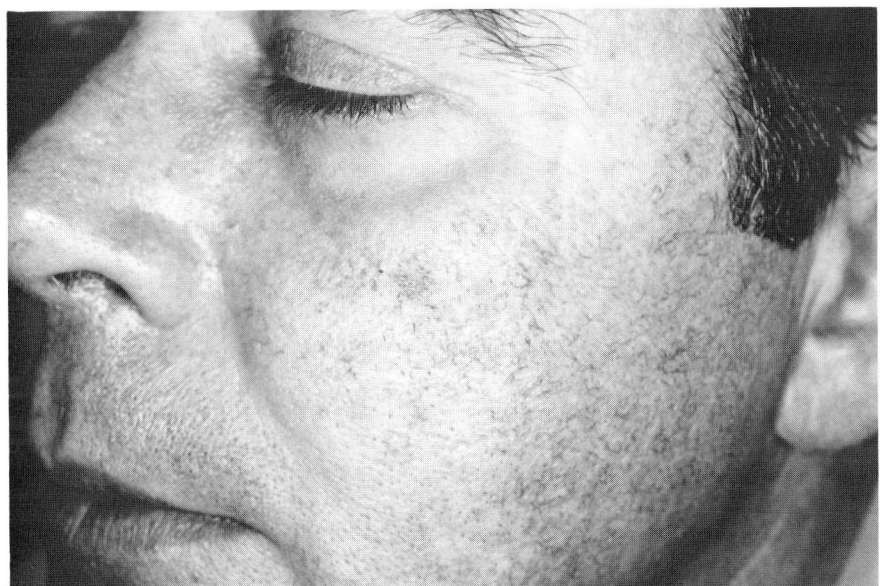

Figure 72. Diffuse telangiectasias of the cheek pretreatment.

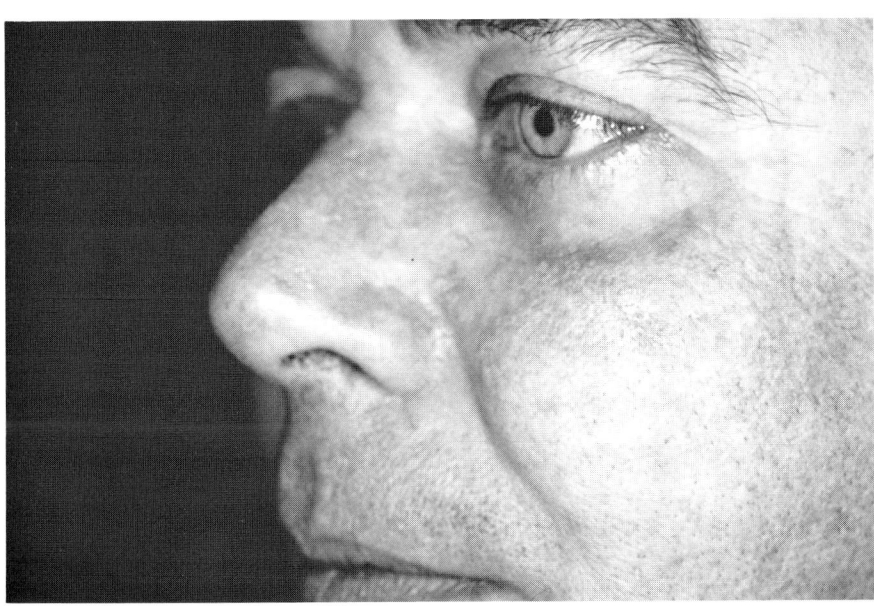

Figure 73. Appearance after treatment of same patient shown in Figure 72.

Figure 74. Preoperative appearance of many telangiectasias on the cheek of a middle-aged woman. (See Figures 75–79.)

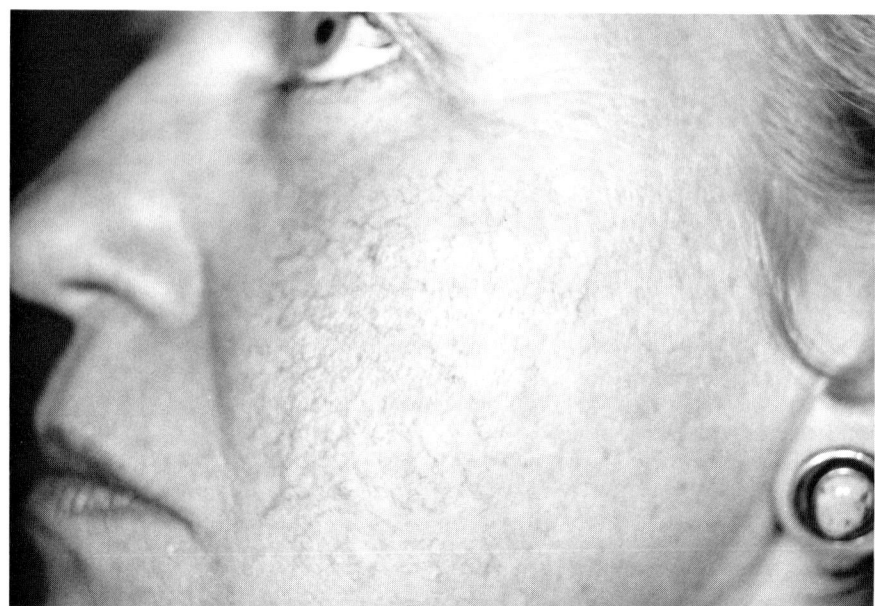

Figure 75. Blush reaction due to the heat of the argon laser which may obscure some small telangiectasias.

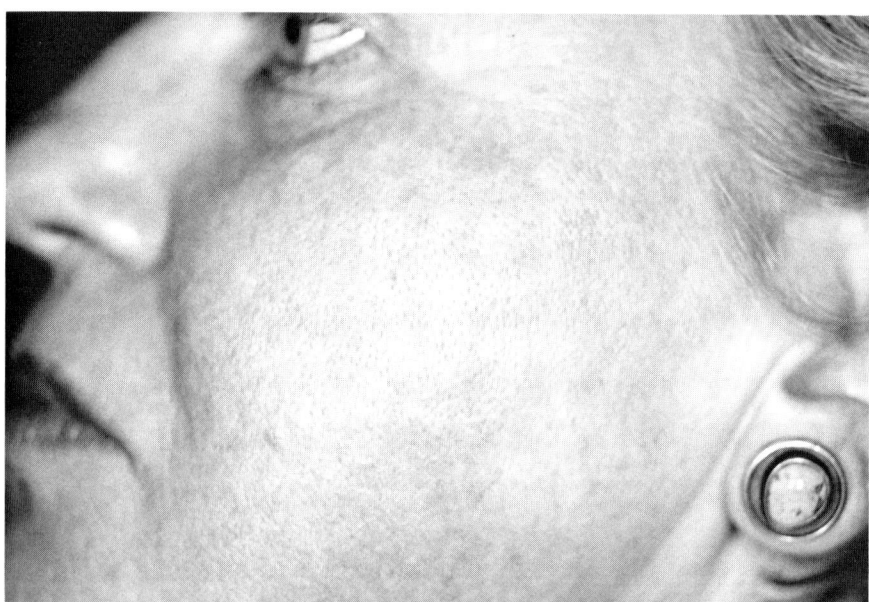

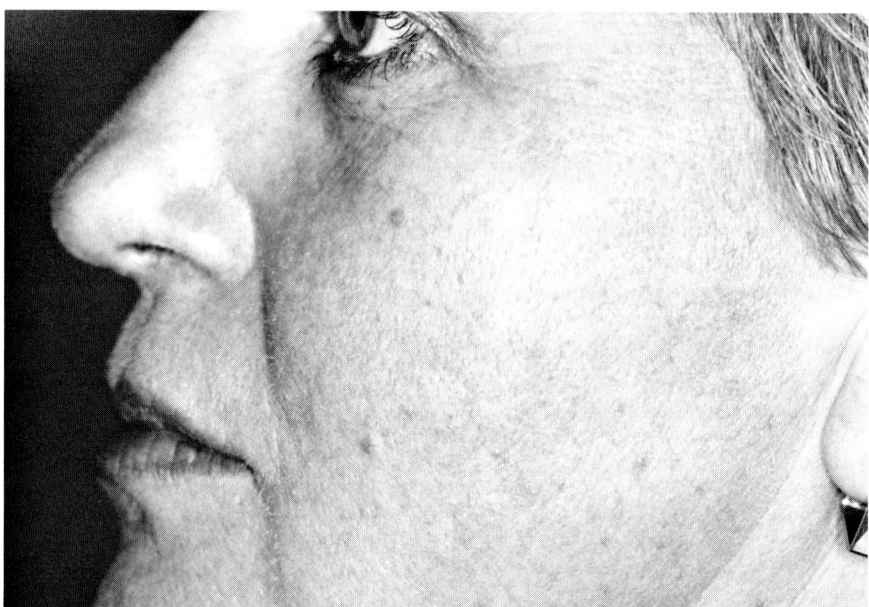

Figure 76. Appearance six weeks after argon laser treatment.

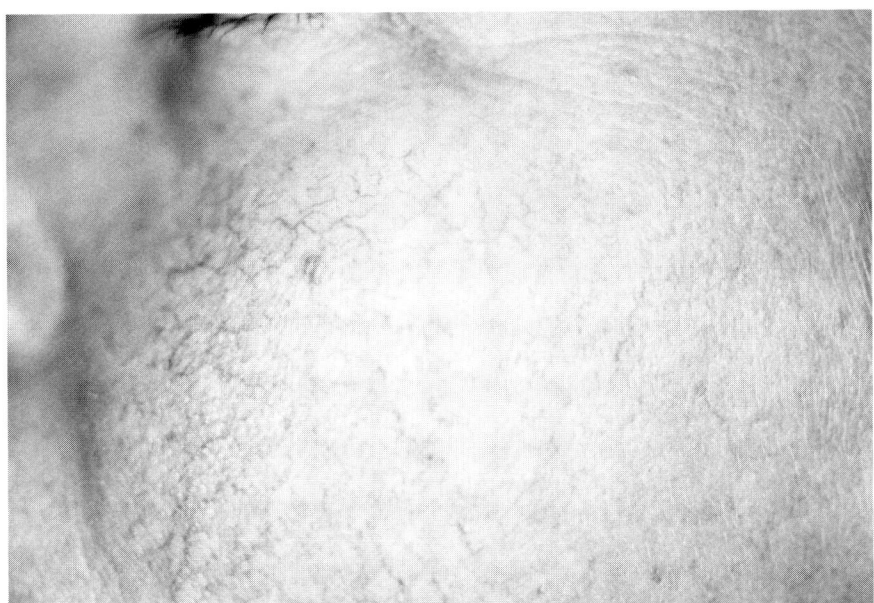

Figure 77. Close-up of patient preoperatively demonstrated in Figure 74.

(Figures 74–79) (see color insert). With these extremely short pulses, most patients can tolerate the mild discomfort associated with this form of therapy without difficulty. Even in the most sensitive patients, if a short pause is given between every three to four pulses during which cooling can occur, the discomfort can be minimized. Since these lesions are often aggravated by emotional stress, spicy foods, alcoholic beverages, as well as heat, the laser may cause some temporary, immediate blushing of the surrounding skin which makes additional treatment impossible since the normal vessels hide the telangiectasias (Figures 80–82) (see color insert). As a consequence, the patient should be told in advance that several treatments may be required in order to satisfactorily treat a large number of vessels. Following laser treatments, most patients will note a small, fine, ashy crust on the skin surface at the site of each laser impact. With cleansing using standard soap and water techniques, this usually resolves completely in three to four days. During this healing period, the use of cosmetics is not suggested. If retreatment ap-

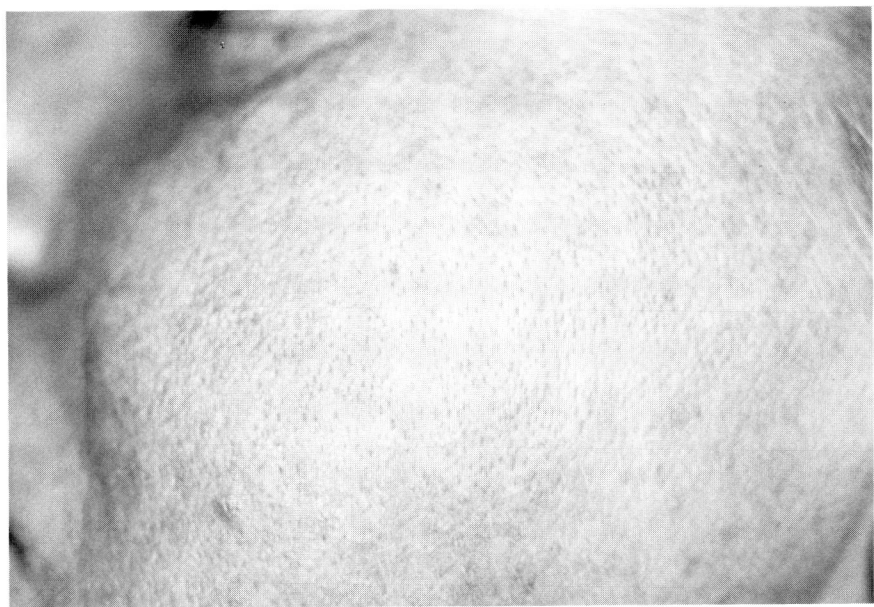

Figure 78. Close-up of patient in Figure 77 showing blush reaction and some focal areas of white discoloration at points of argon laser impact immediately postoperatively.

Figure 79. Final appearance six weeks after argon laser treatment of patient shown in Figure 77.

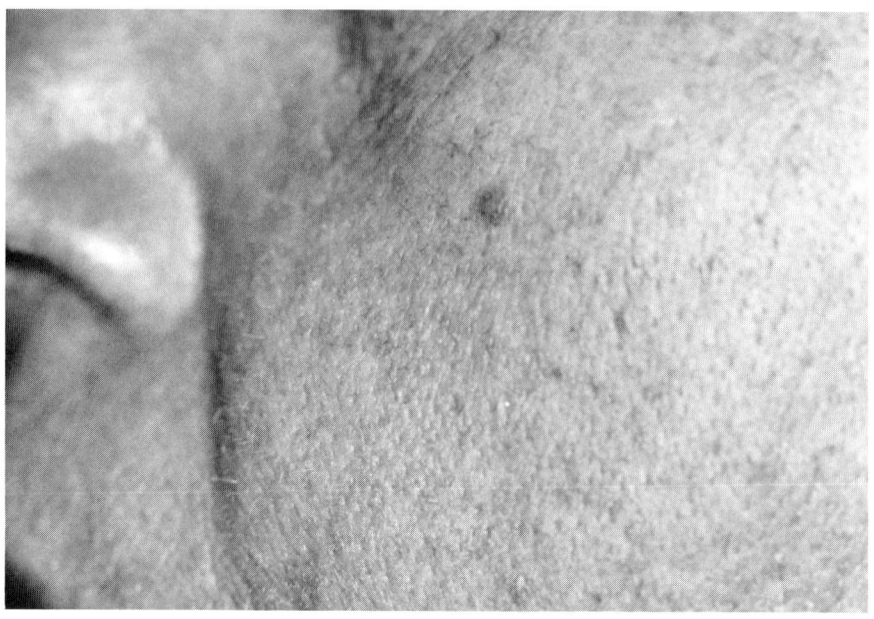

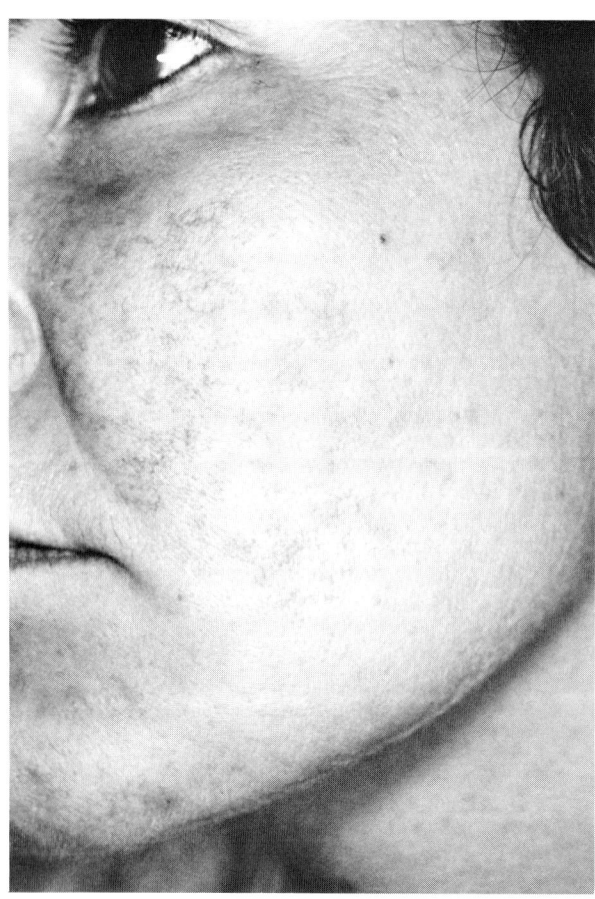

Figure 80. Preoperative appearance of telangiectasias of the cheek.

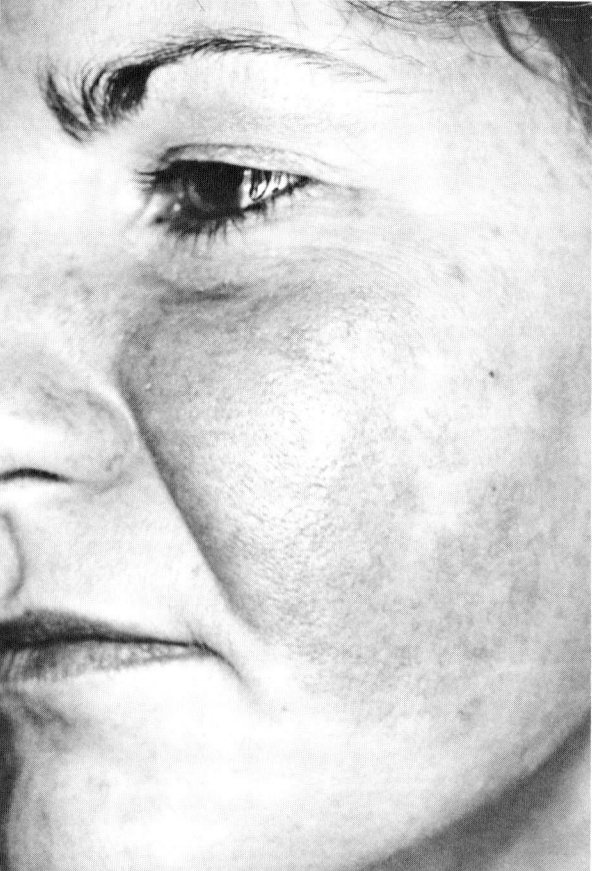

Figure 81. Profound blush reaction after argon laser treatment of patient seen in Figure 80.

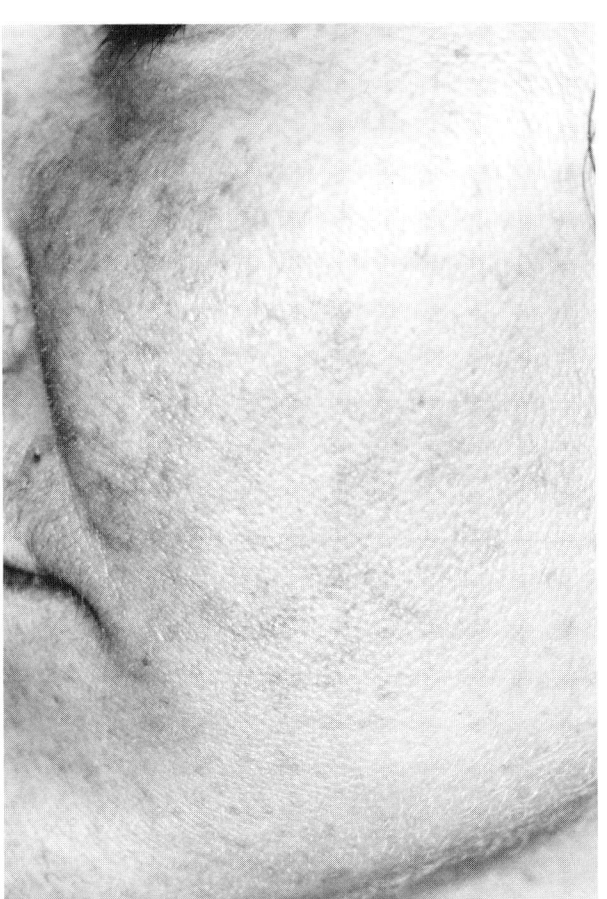

Figure 82. Partial improvement of telangiectasias of patient seen in Figure 80 with persistence of some of the vessels which will require additional treatment.

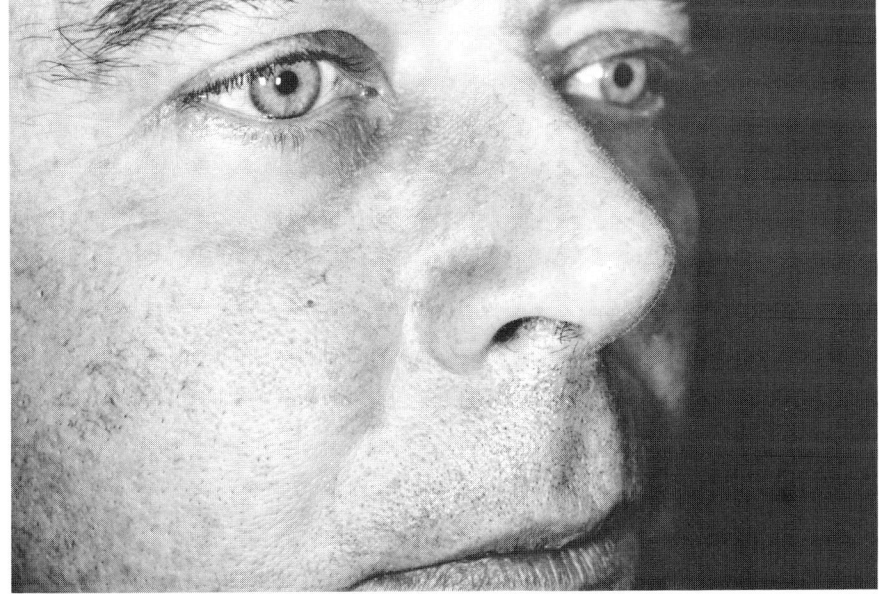

Figure 83. Preoperative appearance of many telangiectasias of the nose.

Figure 84. Appearance of the nose six weeks after argon laser treatment showing almost complete resolution with one treatment session.

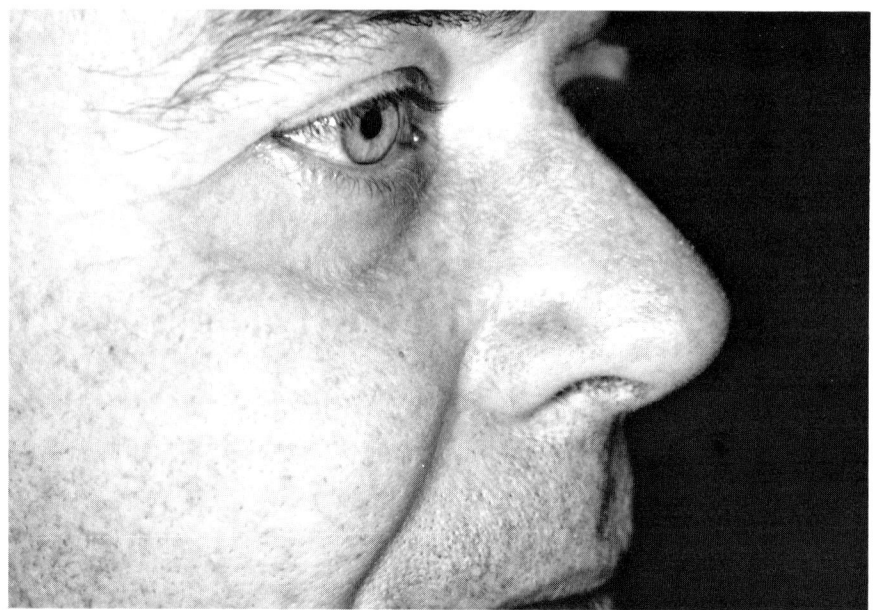

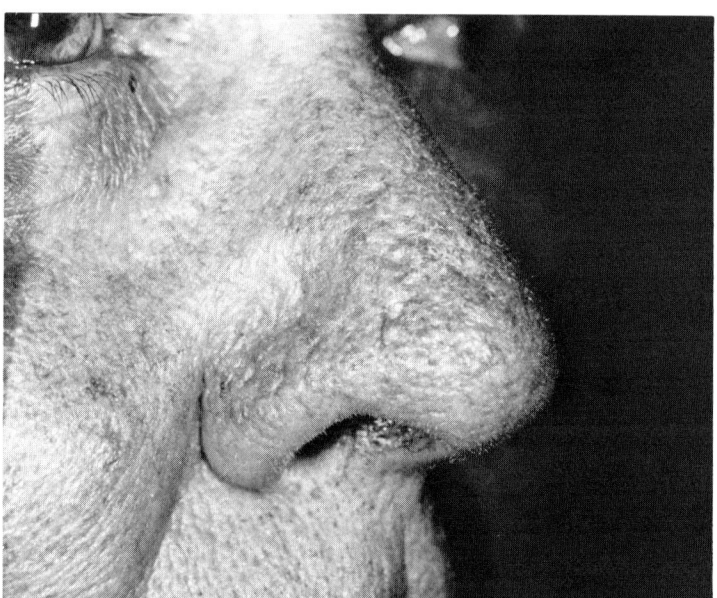

Figure 85. Numerous telangiectasias of the nasal ala and tip preoperatively.

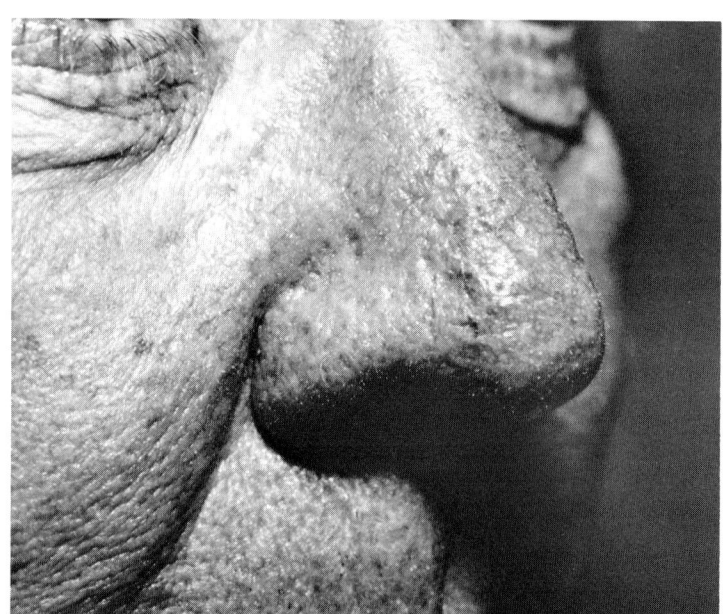

Figure 86. Appearance of patient in Figure 85 six weeks after argon laser treatment showing persistence of some small vessels, but substantial improvement with argon laser treatment.

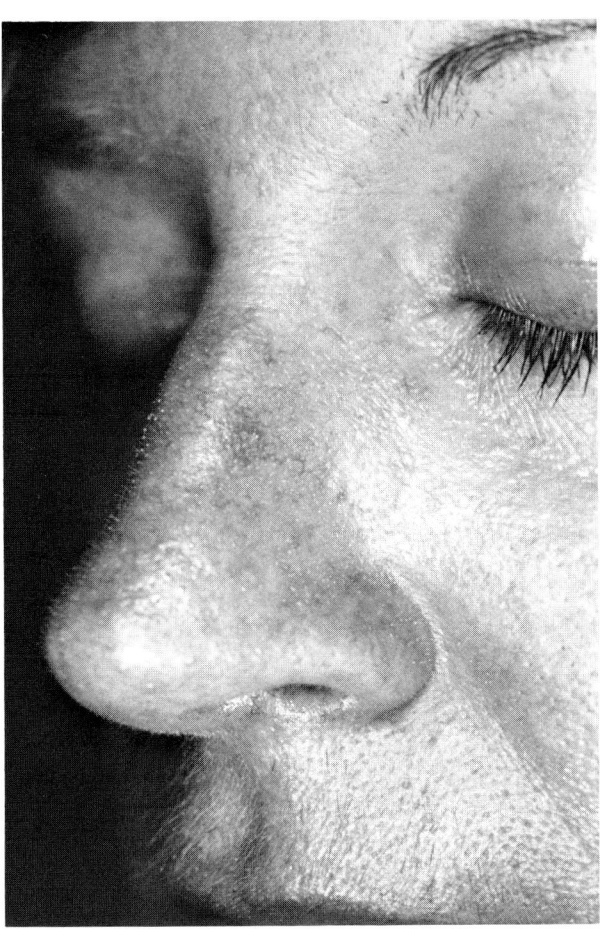

Figure 87. Diffuse as well as focal areas of telangiectasia on the nose preoperatively.

pears to be necessary, this can be safely performed in four to six weeks without difficulty.

Telangiectasias on the nose and perinasal areas are especially common. Treatment with the argon laser can yield excellent results in these patients (Figures 83–88). When treating these types of blood vessels, pulses of laser energy are delivered at points along the length of each vessel until blanching occurs. This may produce a fine white spider-web appearance (Figures 89–94)

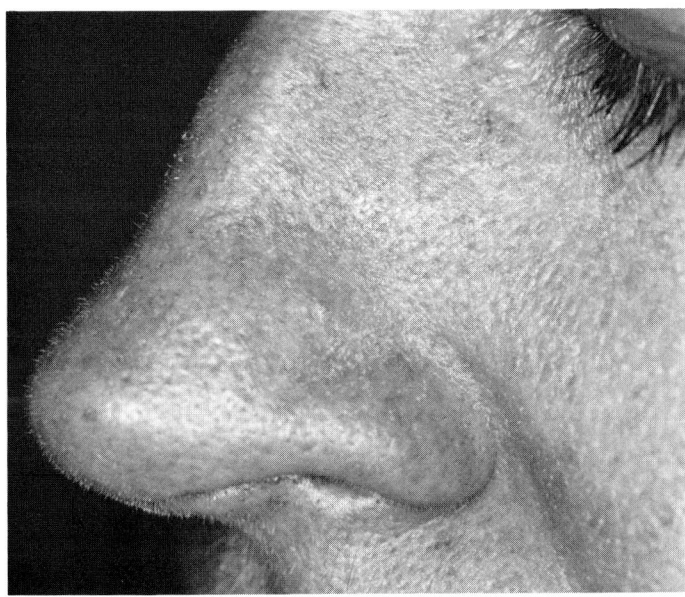

Figure 88. Same patient as in Figure 87 six weeks after argon laser treatment showing approximately 60% improvement with one treatment session using the argon laser.

Figure 89. Preoperative appearance of telangi-ectasias of the nasal bridge and ala.

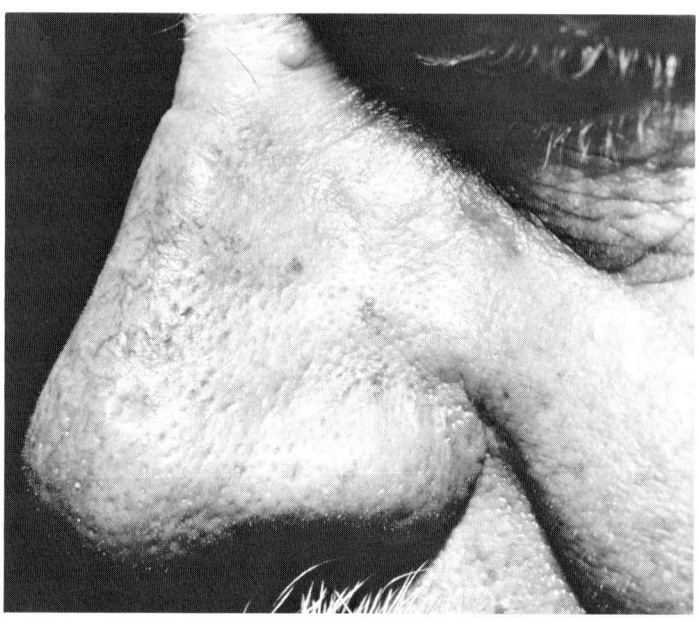

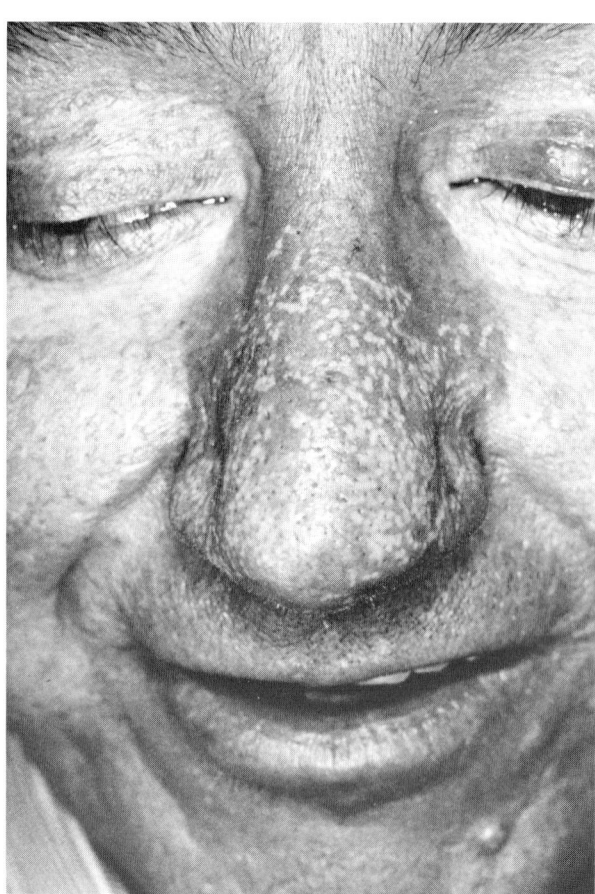

Figure 90. Spiderweb appearance after argon laser treat-ment which is not due to vascular constriction, but rather reflects protein coaguation.

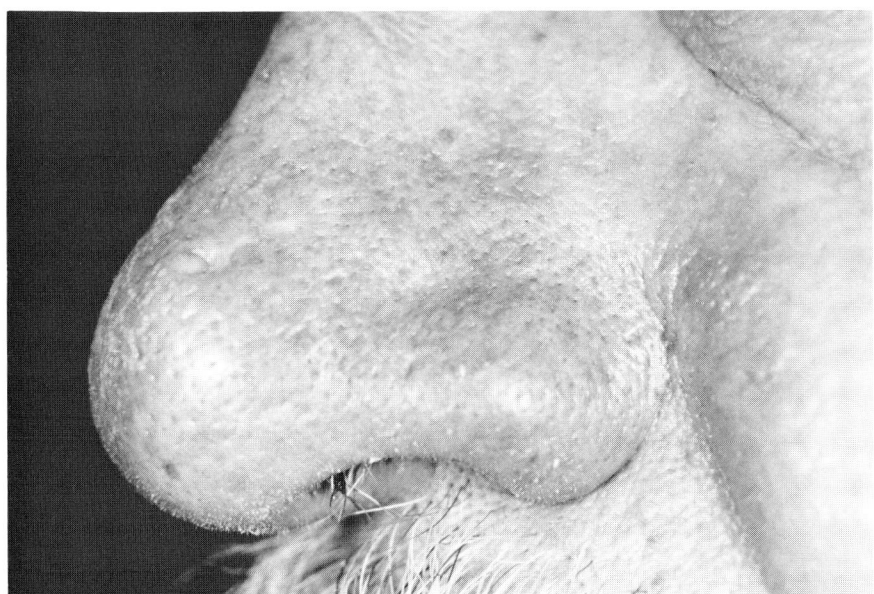

Figure 91. Same patient seen in Figure 89 showing almost complete resolution of telangiectasias of the ala and bridge.

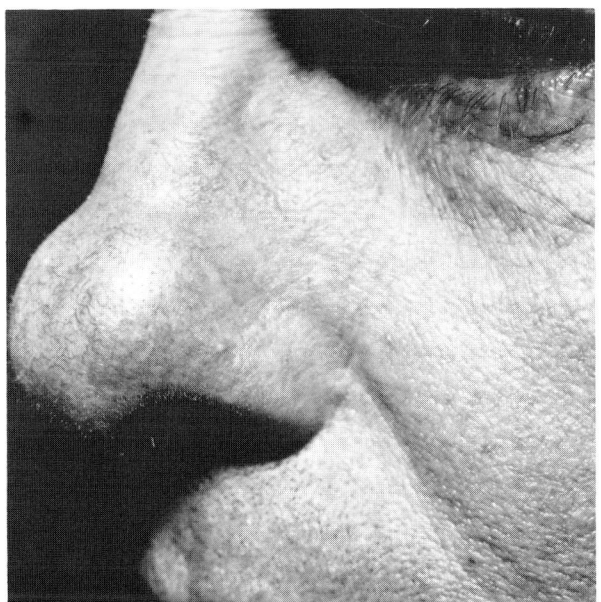

Figure 92. Prominent telangiectasias of the nasal tip and ala preoperatively.

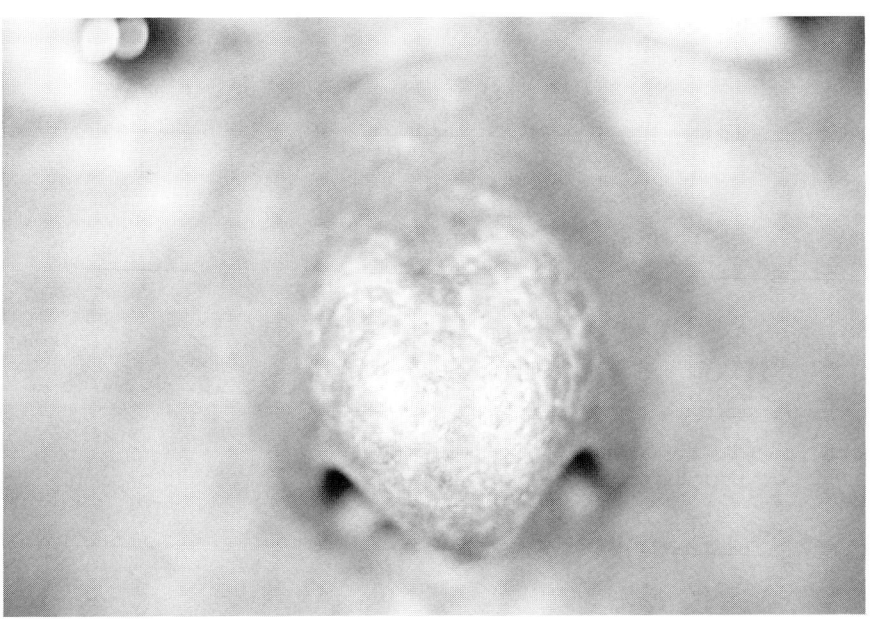

Figure 93. Spiderweb type of white, ashy, argon laser impact points after treatment of patient seen in Figure 92. Again, protein coagulation and not true vascular effects are demonstrated.

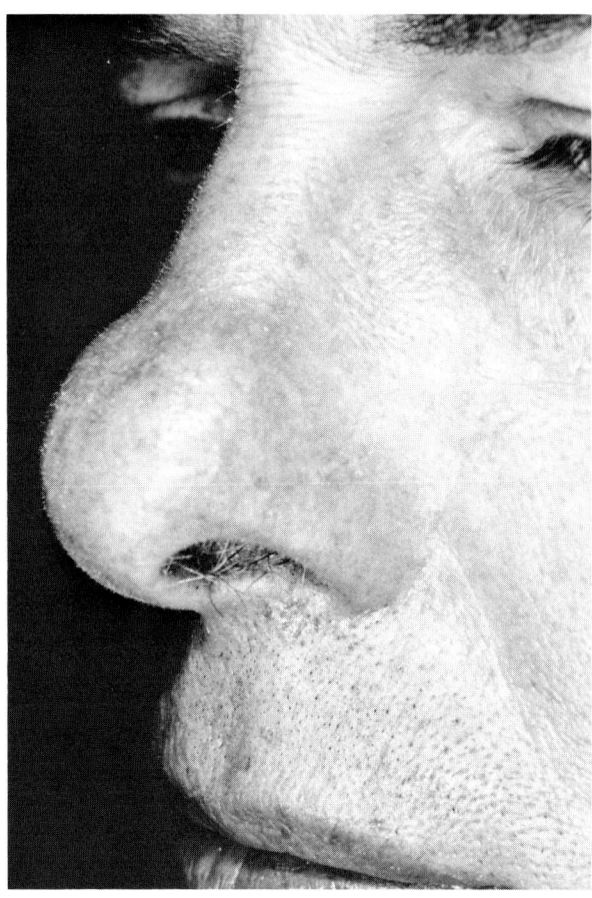

Figure 94. Same patient seen in Figure 92 showing almost complete resolution of telangiectasias of the tip and ala.

immediately after treatment that tends to disappear within 24 hours followed by a slower resolution of the treated vessels over a period of six to 12 weeks.

Hereditary Hemorrhagic Telangiectasia

In the syndrome hereditary hemorrhagic telangiectasia, telangiectasias may develop on the mucous membranes of the lip (Figures 95 and 96) and nasal passages. Because extensive bleeding may occur from these small dilated vessels, treatment may be indicated for more than cosmetic reasons. In these cases, argon laser photocoagulation has proven to be extremely valuable. The vessels in this condition tend to be more mat-like, but through the delivery of a small beam of laser energy to each vessel, they can usually be traced out in their entirety without difficulty. Once again, local anesthesia is not employed, but if discomfort is significant, a small pause between pulses is usually all that is necessary to limit discomfort during treatment.

If these telangiectatic vessels are located on the nasal mucosa, an alotomy may be required (Figure 97) to permit sufficient exposure of the blood vessels so that treatment with the argon laser can proceed (Figure 98). This alotomy can be performed under local anesthesia permitting the alae to be reflected superiorly and to allow precise delivery of argon laser pulses along the length of each telangiectatic blood vessel. Once laser

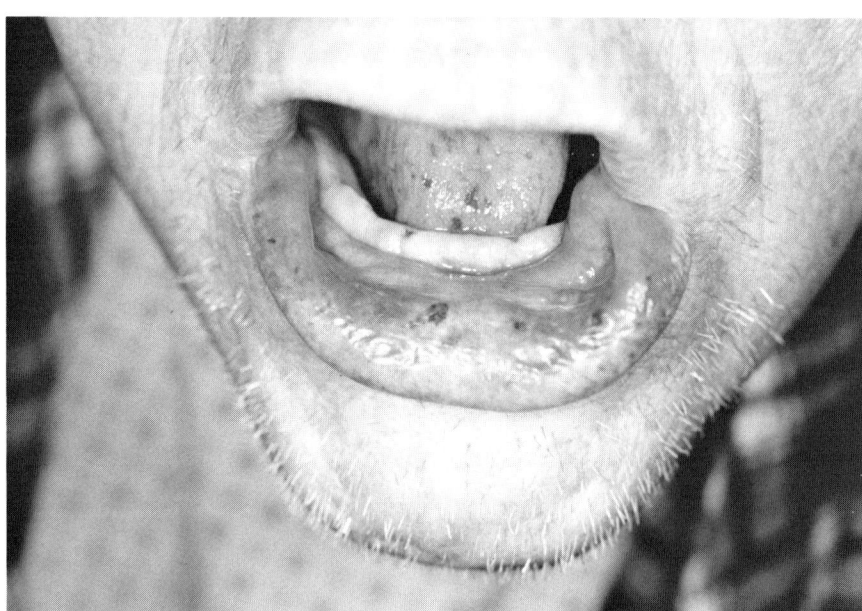

Figure 95. A patient with hereditary hemorrhagic telangiectasia with numerous telangiectasias of the lower lip preoperatively.

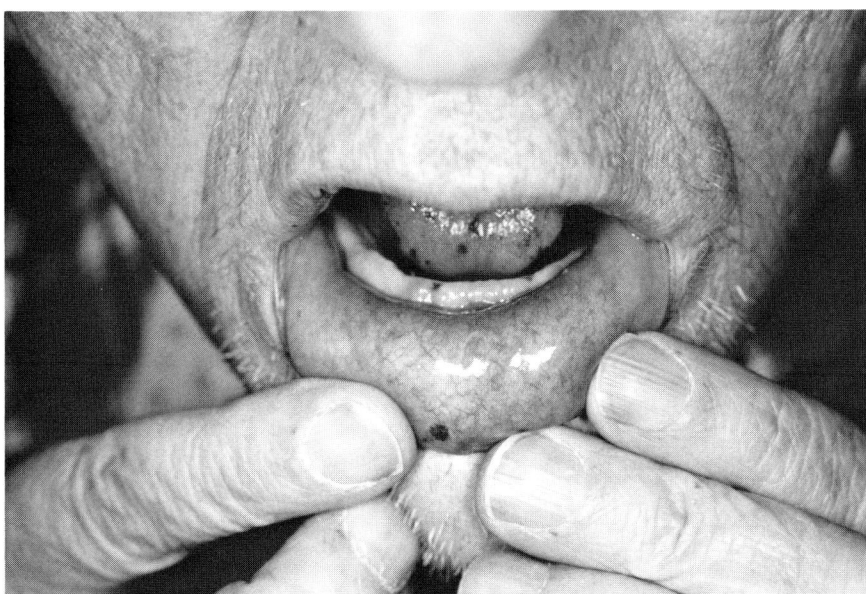

Figure 96. Same patient as in Figure 95 after argon laser treatment showing almost complete resolution of ectatic vessels.

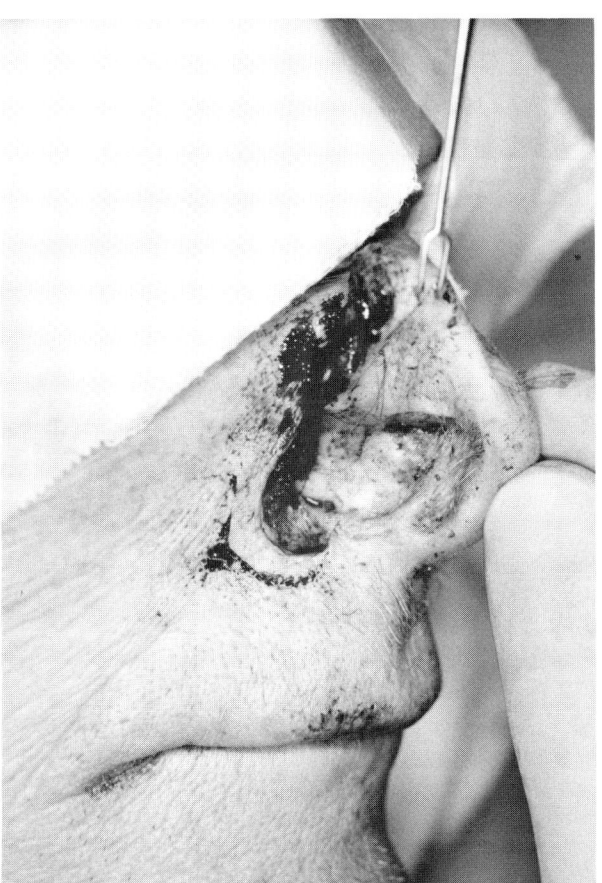

Figure 97. Alatomy has been performed to permit exposure of telangiectatic vessels of the nasal mucosa in a patient with hereditary hemorrhagic telangiectasia.

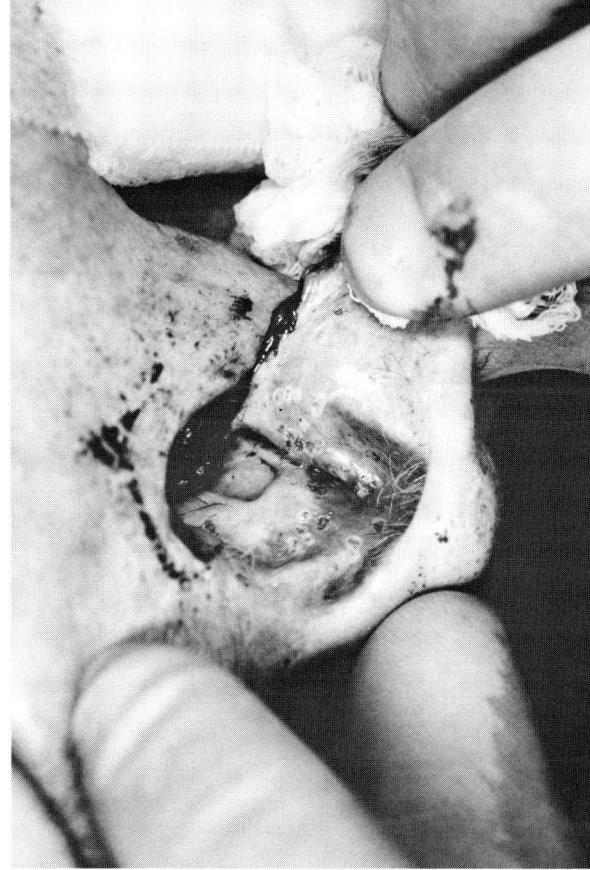

Figure 98. Same patient seen in Figure 97. Small, linear, white areas are points of argon laser impact overlying telangiectatic vessels of nasal mucosa.

Figure 99. Appearance after repair of alatomy of patient shown in Figure 97.

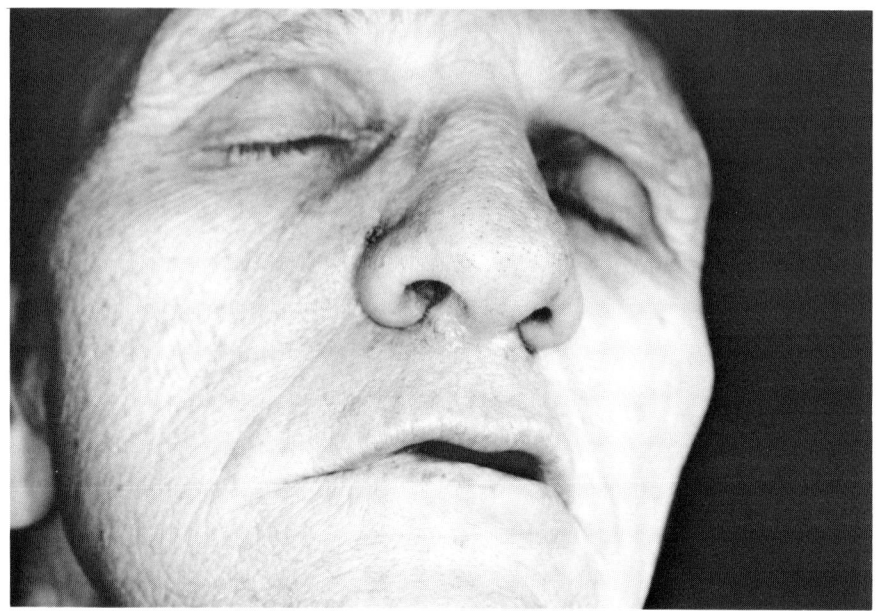

treatment is completed, immediate repair of the alotomy and packing of the nose to prevent any postoperative bleeding from the incision line can be performed (Figure 99).

Spider Angiomas

If the telangiectasias are of the spider angioma type, the initial laser pulse is delivered to the central blood vessel which supplies the re-

mainder of the lesion. Once this has resulted in photocoagulation, the arms radiating from this central point can be photocoagulated by pulsing along their length.

Venous Lakes

Another type of vascular lesion that is present with some regularity on the mucous membranes of the lip is known as a venous lake. These fre-

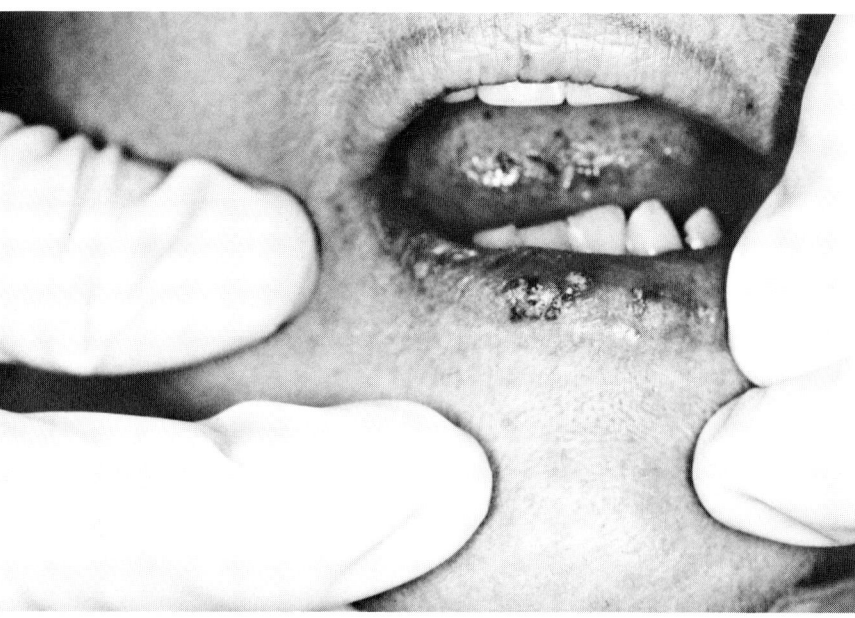

Figure 100. Venous lakes of the lower lip preoperatively.

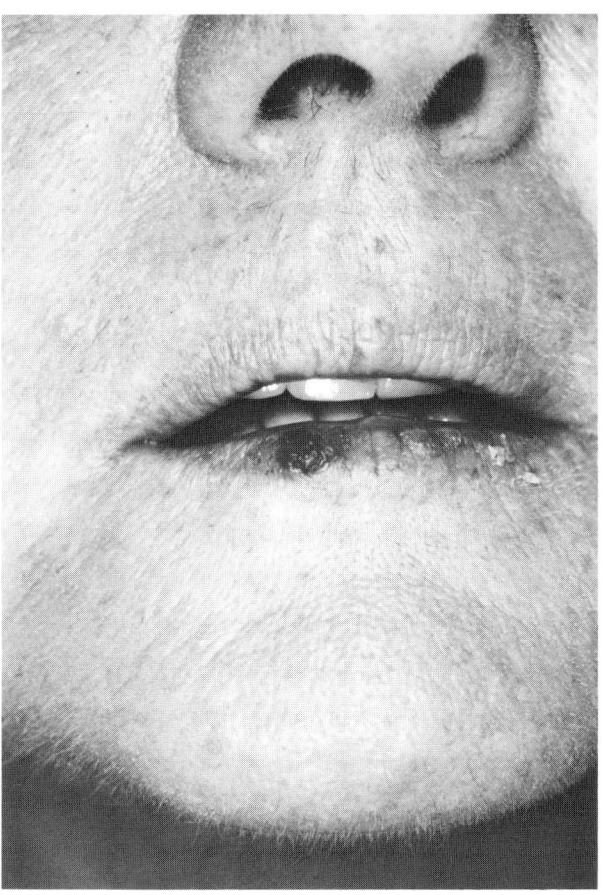

Figure 101. Superficial crusting following argon laser photocoagulation of venous lake for patient seen in Figure 100.

quently multiple, ectatic, 1 to 6 mm, vascular structures (Figure 100) usually form after middle age and are secondary to trauma and chronic sunlight exposure. Because the dilatation of the vascular structures are substantial, venous lakes are subject to bleeding with minor injury. The argon laser has been used to treat these types of lesions with tremendous success. One technique modification that is useful in the treatment of these superficial, but still dilated vascular structures, is to first compress the lesion with a plastic or glass slide and then fire the argon laser through it. By compressing the vascular walls, sufficient thermal energy can usually be delivered to cause damage to the vessel walls (Figure 101) and eventual resolution (Figures 102 and 103). However, if the vessel is treated in its expanded state, the amount of energy delivered may be inadequate to cause thermal injury or resorption. As in all argon laser treatment of vascular structures, there is always a potential for retreatment of some patients. For this reason, each patient should be advised in advance of this so that complete satisfaction can be obtained.

Pyogenic Granuloma

Another condition that only rarely occurs on the face, but that can be successfully treated with

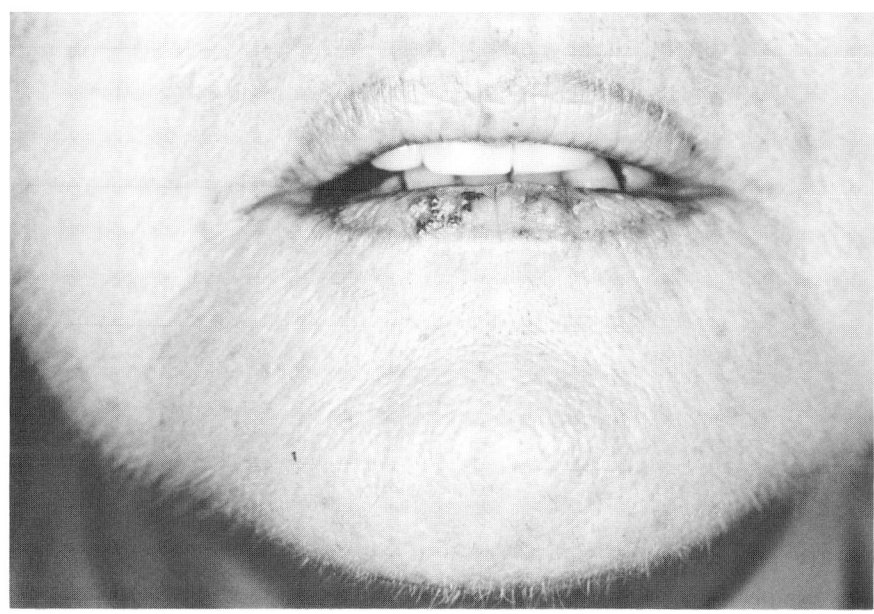

Figure 102. Superficial crusting seen one week post argon laser treatment of patient shown in Figure 100.

Figure 103. Slight xerosis persists, but all vascular elements of the lower lip have resolved ten weeks after argon laser treatment for patient seen in Figure 100.

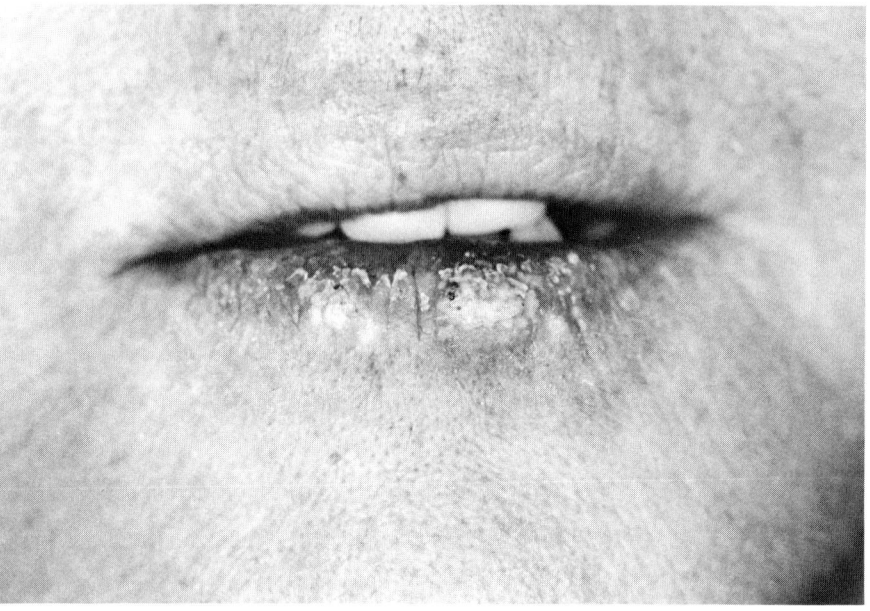

argon laser photocoagulation is the pyogenic granuloma. These vascular lesions tend to occur after minor trauma and represent a proliferation of granulation tissue. By argon laser photocoagulation, the vascular structures can be stimulated to involute. Since spontaneous involution may occur with this lesion, the argon laser is probably only indicated for those resistant lesions or lesions that continue to grow for a substantial period of time. In this situation, the laser treatment parameters are usually based on prior experience with similar lesions on other parts of the body.

However, a pulse duration of 0.10 seconds, 3 watts of power, and a beam size of 1 to 2 mm are the parameters typically used in the treatment of these lesions.

ARGON LASER TREATMENT OF PIGMENTED CUTANEOUS LESIONS

Recognizing that the argon laser emission spectrum overlaps the absorption spectrum for melanin, the laser surgeon can utilize the argon

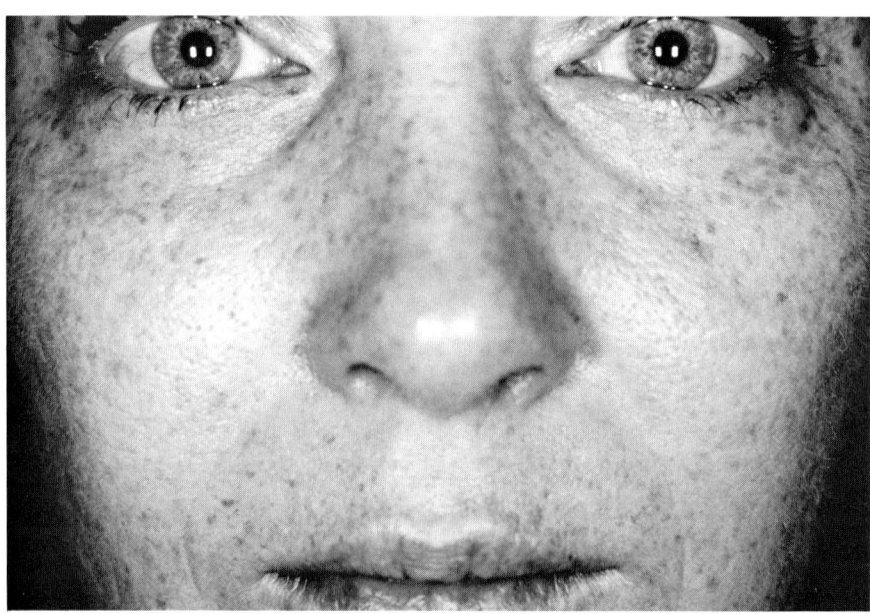

Figure 104. Numerous ephelids of the cheeks preoperatively.

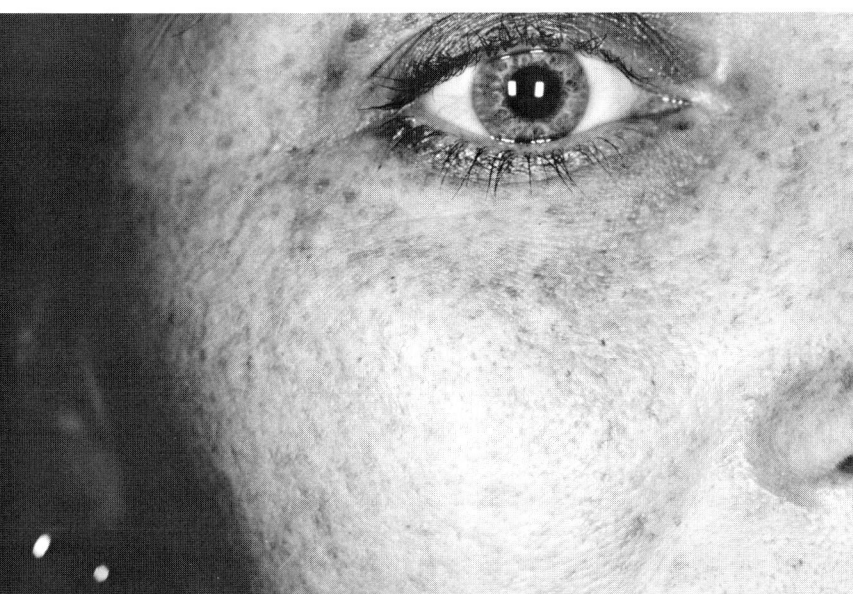

Figure 105. Same patient as in Figure 104 with a decrease in the amount of color of ephelids on the cheek after argon laser therapy.

laser for treatment of pigmented lesions. However, it must be remembered that the type of lesions that are amenable to this form of therapy must be evaluated in advance for possible malignant degeneration. It is inadvisable to treat a suspicious pigmented mole or nevus with the argon laser since histopathologic examination of these types of lesions is recommended. Also, since penetration by the argon laser is relatively superficial, only 1 to 2 mm, this type of treatment is not recommended in the treatment of malignant melanomas, even if they are of the lentigo maligna type, since adequate depth of penetration cannot be guaranteed.

Consequently, the treatment for pigmented lesions of the skin using argon laser photocoagulation is primarily restricted to the treatment of known benign lesions (Table 4). These conditions include the simple lentigo, ephelid (Figures 104 and 105), postinflammatory hyperpigmentation, nevus of Ota, the blue nevus, and granuloma faciale. There may also be some improvement seen in the treatment of chloasma that occurs in the periorbital area after the use of oral contraceptives in females or following pregnancy.

In each of these situations, small test areas are again performed in a similar fashion described for portwine stain angiomas. A series of small test sites are treated with different combinations of time and power. The patient is reexamined six weeks postoperatively to determine whether or not scarring or textural changes have occurred and to evaluate the degree of improvement in

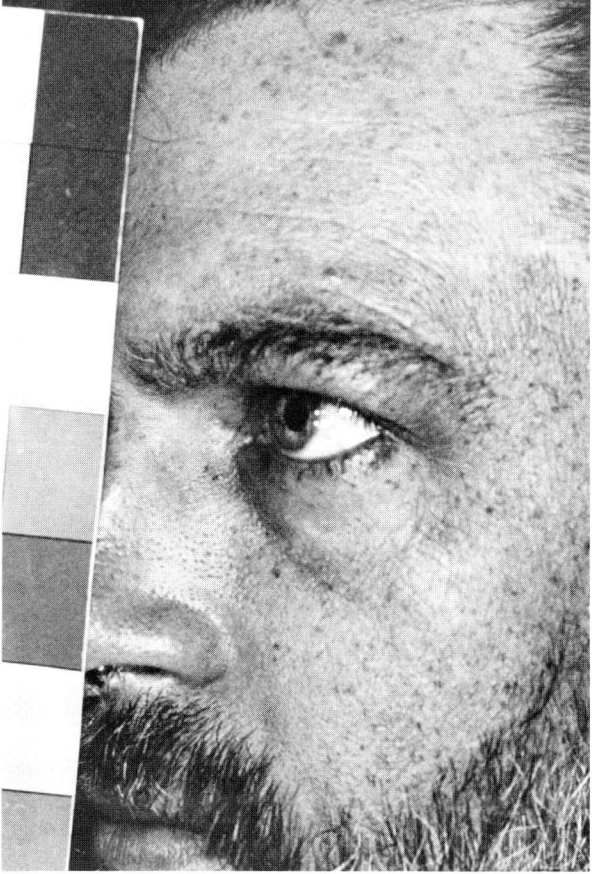

Figure 106. Pigmented nevus (nevus spilus) of the lateral cheek and temple.

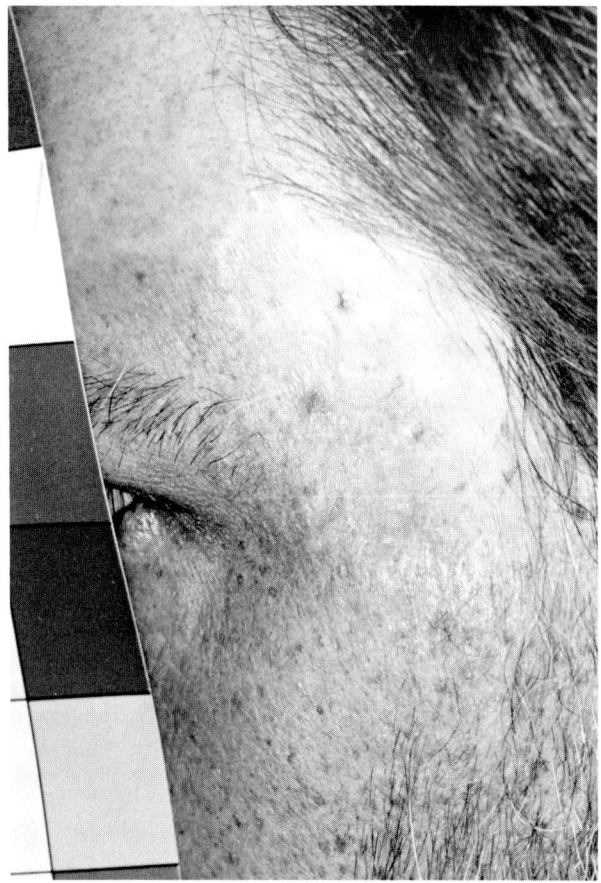

Figure 107. Substantial decrease in the amount of brown pigmentation six weeks after argon laser test treatment has been performed on patient seen in Figure 106.

pigmentation. Once a satisfactory test result has been obtained, the treatment of the remainder of the pigmented lesion can proceed (Figures 106 and 107) accordingly. If the lesion is relatively small, the initial test site may actually result in treatment of the entire lesion, but for larger lesions, test sites are generally recommended.

ARGON LASER EQUIPMENT

The argon laser is relatively less expensive than the carbon dioxide laser. In general, argon lasers can be purchased for between $18,000 and $30,000. There are many new developments in laser technology occurring today that will almost certainly influence the availability of argon laser technology. One of these changes involves the development of a new laser, the dye laser, that can be adjusted in such a way so that it may emit laser energy of many different wavelengths, including the blue-green color range of with the

argon laser. As a consequence, some manufacturers of laser equipment no longer make argon lasers and their availability in the future is not entirely predictable.

One additional consideration that must be kept in mind prior to purchasing argon laser equipment is that water cooling is sometimes required for this rather inefficient laser. The water pressure requirements of the instrument may exceed those of the local regulatory agencies. As a consequence, additional plumbing fixtures or water storage tanks may be required in order for successful operation of the water-cooled argon laser. If the argon laser is air-cooled, additional ventilation may be required in the argon laser operating suite so that the surgeon and patient are not discomforted by use of the equipment. Also, some of the argon lasers manufactured today require three-phase electrical current which may require additional special wiring of the laser operating suite to provide the necessary electricity.

The special eye protection required for safe operation of the argon laser must also be purchased. These glasses cost from $35 up to $200 each and should also be included in determining the initial expense budget for operating an argon laser. The eyeshields that are sometimes used for periorbital or eyelid procedures cost from $12 to $80 each. All of these items are readily available through a variety of different laser equipment manufacturers, but their expense must be included when considering the potential financial benefits of a purchase of an argon laser system.

BIBLIOGRAPHY

Apfelberg DB, Maser MR, Lash H: Argon laser management of cutaneous vascular deformities. West J Med 124:99–101, 1976.

Apfelberg DB, Maser MR, Lash H: Argon laser treatment of cutaneous vascular abnormalities: Progress report. Ann Plast Surg 1:14–18, 1978.

Apfelberg DB, Maser MR, Lash H: Treatment of nevi aranei by means of an argon laser. J Dermatol Surg Oncol 4:172–173, 1978.

Apfelberg DB, Maser MR, Lash H: Argon laser treatment of decorative tattoos. Br J Plast Surg 32:141–144, 1979.

Apfelberg DB, Kosek J, Maser MR, et al: Histology of portwine stains following argon laser treatment. Br J Plast Surg 32:232–237, 1979.

Apfelberg DB, Maser MR, Lash H, et al: The argon laser for cutaneous lesions. JAMA 245:2073–2075, 1981.

Apfelberg D, Greene R, Maser M, et al: Results of argon laser exposure of capillary hemangiomas of infancy — preliminary report. Plast Reconstr Surg 67:188–193, 1981.

Apfelberg DB, Maser MR, Lash H, et al: The role of the argon laser in the management of hemangiomas. Internat J Dermatol 21:579–589, 1982.

Apfelberg DB, Flores JT, Maser MR, et al: Analysis of complications of argon laser treatment for portwine hemangiomas with reference to striped techniques. Lasers Surg Med 2:357–371, 1983.

Apfelberg DB, Maser MR, Lash H, et al: Expanded role of the argon laser in plastic surgery. J Dermatol Surg Oncol 9:145–151, 1983.

Arndt K: Adenoma sebaceum: Successful treatment with argon laser. Plast Reconstr Surg 70:91–93, 1982.

Arndt KA: Argon laser therapy of small cutaneous vascular lesions. Arch Dermatol 118:220–224, 1982.

Arndt KA: Argon laser treatment of lentigo maligna. J Am Acad Dermatol 10:953–957, 1984.

Brauner GJ, Schliftman A: Laser surgery for children. J Dermatol Surg Oncol 13:178–186, 1987.

Cosman B: Experience in the argon laser therapy of portwine stains. Plast Reconstr Surg 65:119–129, 1980.

Dixon JA, Rotering RH, Huether SE: Patient's evaluation of argon laser therapy of portwine stain, decorative tattoo, and essential telangiectasia. Lasers Surg Med 4:181–190, 1984.

Dixon JA, Heuther S, Rotering R: Hypertrophic scarring in argon laser treatment of portwine stains. Plast Reconstr Surg 73:771–777, 1984.

Goldman L, Dreffer R, Rockwell RJ, et al: Treatment of portwine marks by an argon laser. J Dermatol Surg 2:385–388, 1976.

Goldman L, Dreffer R: Laser treatment of extensive mixed cavernous and portwine stains. Arch Dermatol 113:504–505, 1977.

Goldman L: Laser treatment of multiple progressive glomangiomas. Arch Dermatol 114:1853–1854, 1978.

Goldman L: The argon laser and the portwine stain. Plast Reconstr Surg 65:137–139, 1980.

Henderson DL, Cromwell TA, Mes LG: Argon and carbon dioxide laser treatment of hypertrophic and keloid scars. Lasers Surg Med 3:271–277, 1984.

Hobby L: Further evaluation of the potential of the argon laser in the treatment of strawberry hemangiomas. Plast Reconstr Surg 71:481–485, 1983.

Hulsbergen Henning JP, van Gemert MJC: Rhinophyma treated with argon laser. Lasers Surg Med 2:211–215, 1983.

Landthaler M, Haina D, Waidelich W, et al: A three-year experience with the argon laser in dermatotherapy. J Dermatol Surg Oncol 10:456–461, 1984.

Landthaler M, Haina D, Waidelich W, et al: Laser therapy of venous lakes (Bean-Walsh) and telangiectasias. Plast Reconstr Surg 73:78–83, 1984.

Landthaler M, Haina D, Waidelich W, et al: Argon laser therapy of verrucous nevi. Plast Reconstr Surg 74:108–113, 1984.

Lyons GD, Owens RE, Mouney DF: Argon laser destruction of cutaneous telangiectatic lesions. Laryngoscope 91:1322–1325, 1981.

McBurney EI, Leonard GL: Argon laser treatment of portwine hemangiomas: Clinical and histologic correlation. South Med J 74:925–926, 1981.

Noe J, Barsky S, Geer D, et al: Portwine stains and the response to argon laser therapy: Successful treatment and the predictive role of color, age and biopsy. Plast Reconstr Surg 65:130–136, 1980.

Noe JM, Finley J, Rosen S, et al: Postrhinoplasty "red nose":Differential diagnosis and treatment by laser. Plast Reconstr Surg 67:661–664, 1981.

Ohshiro T, Maruyama Y, Nakajima H, et al: Treatment of pigmentation of the lips and oral mucosa in Peutz-Jeghers' syndrome using ruby and argon lasers. Br J Plast Surg 33:346–349, 1980.

Touquet VLR, Carruth JAS: Review of the treatment of portwine stains with the argon laser. Lasers Surg Med 4:191–199, 1984.

Wheeland RG, Kantor GR, Bailin PL, et al: Role of the argon laser in treatment of lymphocytoma cutis. J Am Acad Dermatol 14:267–272, 1986.

3   An Introduction to Carbon Dioxide Laser Surgery

Of all the various laser systems used by medical specialists around the world, the carbon dioxide laser is the one employed most frequently. It is used most often for laser treatment of lesions on the head and neck as well. The versatility of this laser system is due to its two distinctly different modes of operation (Figures 108 and 109). The mid-infrared, invisible, carbon dioxide laser energy of 10,600 nm, can be utilized when focused to an extremely small beam to incise tissues. It can also be used with its beam of energy broadened or defocused to vaporize tissue. Each of these two different modes of operations permits the laser surgeon to perform entirely different types of surgery with this instrument.

The carbon dioxide laser energy is developed within an optical cavity containing a mixture of three different gases: one part carbon dioxide, one and one-half parts nitrogen, and four parts helium (Table 5). The energy from this relatively efficient laser (10–15%) is delivered to the target tissue through sealed tubes (Figures 110 and 111) and angled articulating mirrored joints to a movable handpiece (Figure 112) that has a built-in focusing lens. For precise energy delivery, all carbon dioxide laser systems employ coaxial, red light beams generated by helium-neon lasers. This aiming beam is, therefore, an integral part of the carbon dioxide laser system, allowing accurate delivery of the otherwise invisible carbon dioxide laser energy.

The energy of the carbon dioxide laser is absorbed nonselectively by all types and colors of living soft tissues since there is no chromophore for this wavelength of laser light. Instead, the minimum scatter that occurs in soft tissue is not due to absorption by a chromophore of the skin or mucous membrane, but rather by absorption by intracellular and extracellular water. In this way, total absorption of the carbon dioxide laser energy occurs in 0.1 mm of soft tissue, since it is composed of 80% to 90% water.

SAFETY PROCEDURES REQUIRED FOR THE CARBON DIOXIDE LASER

The carbon dioxide laser has its own set of potential risks when it is employed in the treatment of any medical condition. One of the greatest hazards associated with use of this laser is the possibility of ignition of surgical drapes, clothing, or flammable substances. When this laser energy strikes tissue, it converts intracellular or extracellular water immediately to steam and smoke at 100°C. When performing conventional, non-laser surgical procedures, sterilized cotton or synthetic materials are used as operating drapes and are placed around the operative site to minimize the risk of potential contamination from the surrounding tissue. If the carbon dioxide laser beam should accidentally be directed onto one of these dry, surgical drapes, ignition may occur.

A simple method to minimize this potential risk is to apply sterile water or sterile saline to the surgical drapes (Figure 113) surrounding the operative field prior to beginning the surgical procedure. In this way, if the carbon dioxide laser beam should come in contact with the operating drapes, the energy from the laser beam would be absorbed by the water in them and be converted into steam and heat without ignition. A newly developed sterile operating drape has recently been developed that is resistant to ignition from contact with the laser beam and at the same time does not require preoperative soaking of the material for safety.

The possible ignition of other flammable substances found in the laser operating room is another commonly overlooked source of potential hazard. It is for that reason that all flammable materials should be excluded from the laser suite to prevent the accidental or inadvertent use at the time of laser surgery. All preoperative prepping solutions that contains alcohol, such as isopropyl

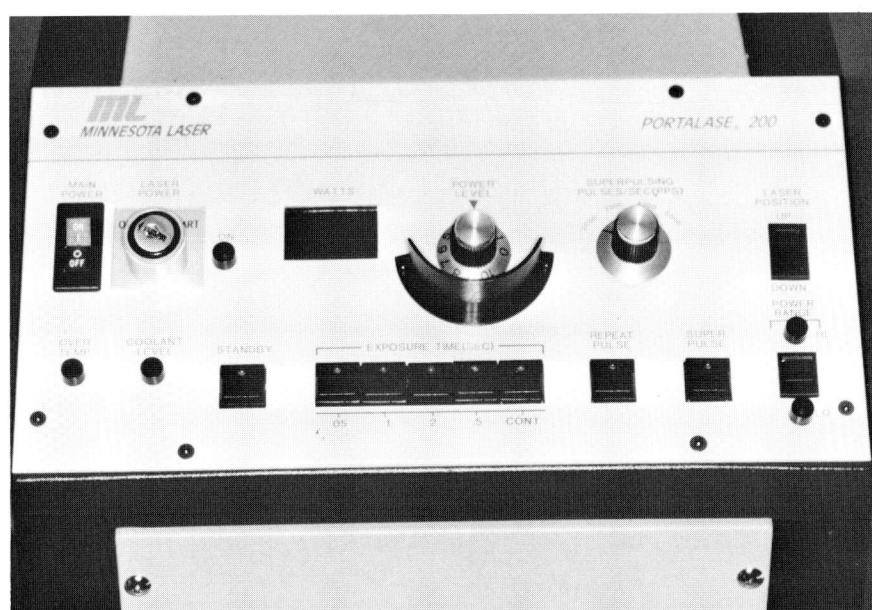

Figure 122. The control panel of a standard carbon dioxide laser showing the various switches and dials that must be used for proper operation.

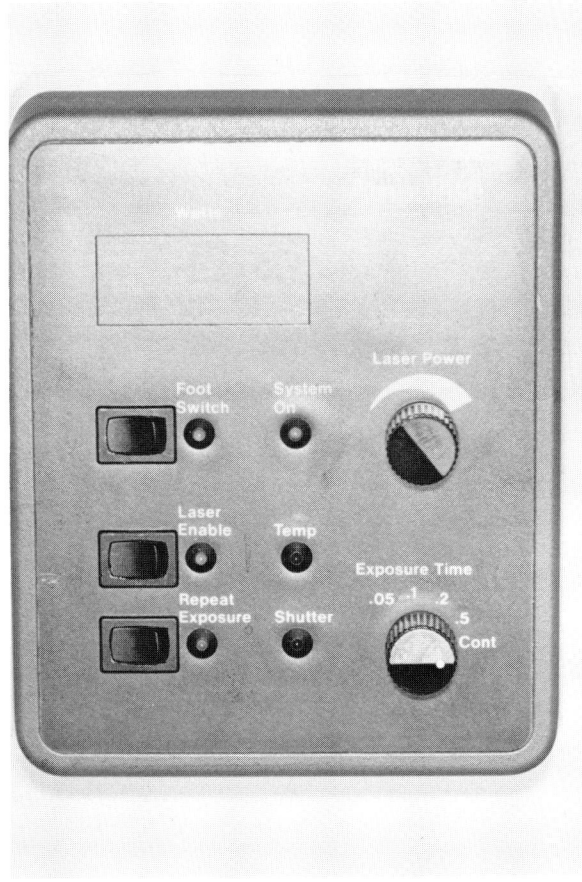

Figure 123. Carbon dioxide laser control panel.

dioxide laser energy to it. If the instrument is properly aligned and the helium-neon laser is coaxial with the carbon dioxide laser beam, the carbon dioxide laser energy should strike the target precisely where it is being illuminated by the helium-neon laser beam. The box-like safety housing that protects the foot pedal from accidentally being activated should also be checked for secure attachment (Figure 125).

As with all laser procedures, a laser safety sign should be placed on the door to the entrance to the laser operating room. This warning sign should state that a laser is in use and the wavelength of the laser light being employed should be listed. The door to the laser room should be closed and in some cases locked if the laser operating suite is in a high-traffic area. Since the carbon dioxide laser energy will not pass through plastic or glass, if the laser operating room has an exterior window, these windows need not be covered during the laser procedure since passage through them will not occur.

If working in the immediate vicinity of the eye, many laser surgeons recommend use of special polished, stainless steel scleral eyeshields. This is similar in design and function to the eyeshields discussed in argon laser phototherapy, but this kind of shield will reflect the carbon dioxide laser energy and cause it to diverge without causing injury to the surrounding tissues. It would require a tremendous amount of carelessness or inattention for the stainless steel eyeshield (see Figure 47) to become sufficiently heated by con-

Figure 124. Carbon dioxide laser control panel.

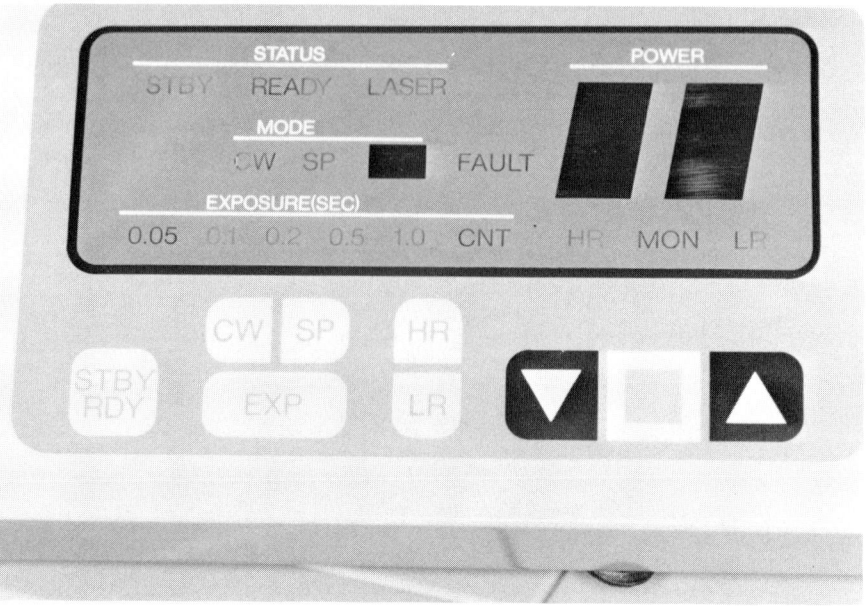

tact with the carbon dioxide laser beam to cause thermal injury to the eye. However, the plastic or methylmethacrylate eyeshield may, indeed, become hot or even melt if prolonged contact with the carbon dioxide laser beam occurs. If not working in the periorbital area, the simplest way to minimize risk of injury to the eyes is to apply wet, cotton gauzes to the eyelids and hold them in place with plastic or polycarbonate goggles.

CARBON DIOXIDE LASER EQUIPMENT

The cost of the various carbon dioxide laser systems generally varies with the amount of power each laser is able to produce. A laser with a maximum power to tissue of 20 watts will cost in the range of $25,000 to $50,000. Carbon dioxide lasers with a maximum power of 100 watts often

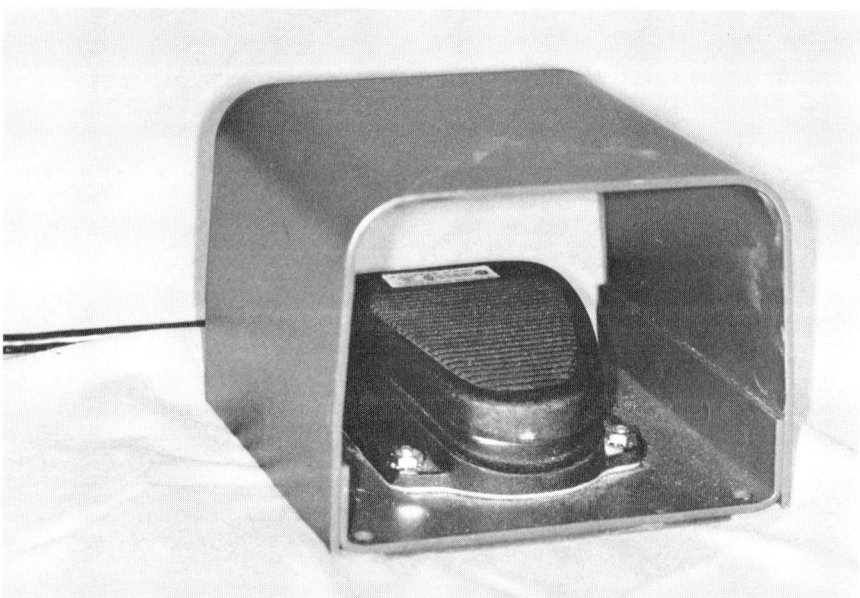

Figure 125. Protective metal housing encloses the carbon dioxide laser foot pedal activating switch.

sociated with movement of these large gas cylinders and has also made the carbon dioxide laser more portable. Most of the current carbon dioxide lasers in use today require no special electrical wiring and can be plugged into standard operating room outlets without difficulties. The carbon dioxide laser, however, can generate a modest amount of heat and as a consequence many of the laser operating rooms are equipped with special cooling systems to aid in the ventilation of the operating room.

One cost that cannot be overlooked in the purchasing of carbon dioxide laser technology is that of the smoke evacuator. This vital instrument, which is not only necessary for the safe operation of the laser but also for the more pleasant surgery by removal of noxious gases from the environment, may cost anywhere from $1200 to $3500. These evacuators can be relatively small, hand-carried instruments (Figures 116 and 117) with limited function, or can be large desk-sized pieces of equipment (Figure 115) that can be

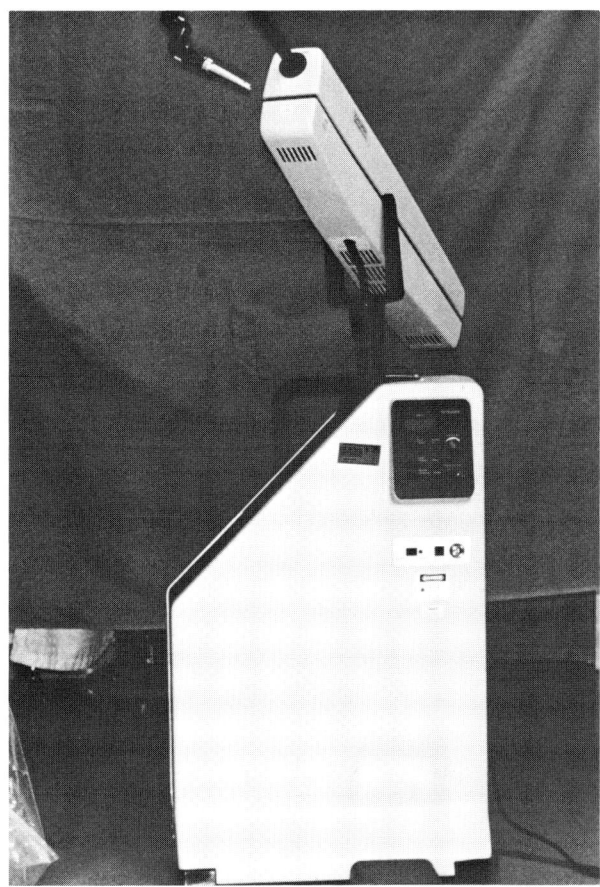

Figure 126. One of the new sealed-tube carbon dioxide laser units.

cost in excess of $100,000. One of the new technologies in carbon dioxide laser surgery is the super-pulse laser. This type of laser system is capable of delivering extremely high laser energy in extremely short, millisecond pulses. As consequence of the high energy required for this type of technology, these instruments may cost between $40,000 and $100,000.

Another of the recent advances in carbon dioxide laser technology has been the development of sealed-tube technology (Figure 126) which eliminates the need for flow-through gases (Figure 127). Most of the original carbon dioxide lasers required a mixture of carbon dioxide, helium, and nitrogen gases to be continuously infused into the laser chamber for the generation of the laser beam to occur. This required placement of large cylinders of these gases in each laser suite for operation of the carbon dioxide laser.

The new technology now permits the creation of carbon dioxide laser energy without the need for these supplemental sources of gases. This helps to eliminate the hazards and confusion as-

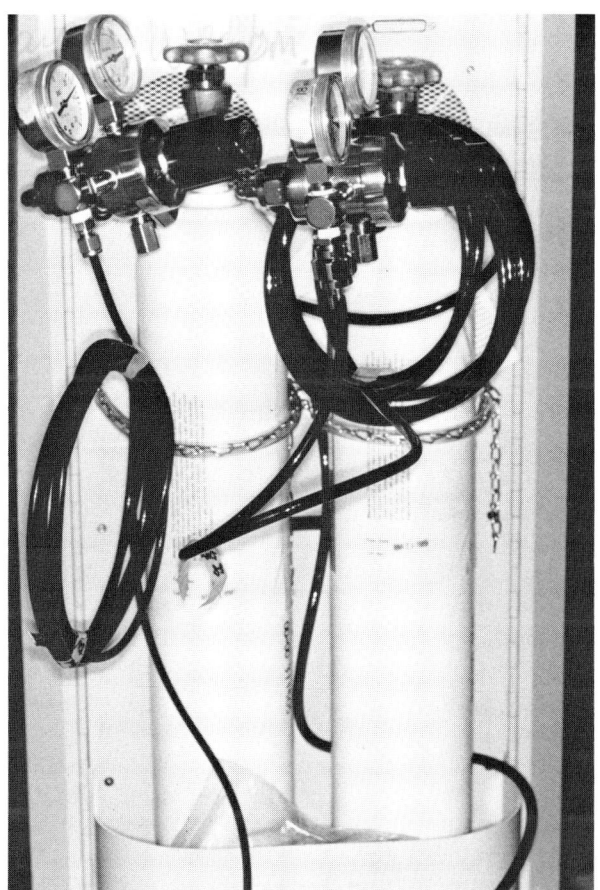

Figure 127. Gas tanks used for flow-through carbon dioxide laser units.

used as surgical instrument trays. These added hidden expenses must be included when considering purchase of a carbon dioxide laser.

ADVANTAGES OF CARBON DIOXIDE SURGERY

The prime benefit in use of the carbon dioxide laser relates to the precision with which it can be delivered to the target tissue. A single pulse of carbon dioxide laser will penetrate no more than 0.10 mm into soft tissue and at the same time cause only limited spread of thermal energy into the surrounding tissue. This minimizes the amount of potential harm that can be done to tissue surrounding a given lesion or tumor. As a consequence, rapid healing will likely occur in most cases without any additional precautions or maneuvers required.

The second major benefit of carbon dioxide laser surgery relates to the effects of the thermal energy that is created following absorption of carbon dioxide laser energy by soft tissues. This heat will cause sealing of small vascular channels of 0.5 to 1.5 mm in diameter with great predictability. Not only does this provide the surgeon with greater visibility during surgery, it minimizes blood loss and may make the patient feel more comfortable during the surgical procedure, especially if it is being performed under local anesthesia.

At the same time that the carbon dioxide laser seals small vascular channels, it also seals lymphatic channels. This potential benefit of the carbon dioxide laser in oncologic surgery has yet to be proven, but at least theoretically, the sealing of lymphatics might convey an advantage to the patient suffering from a cutaneous or mucous membrane malignancy that is capable of metastasis, like melanoma or squamous-cell carcinoma. Also, the sensory nerve endings of skin and mucous membranes are sealed as they contact the carbon dioxide laser beam. For this reason, in most bilaterally compared surgical cases, laser-treated sites are associated with less discomfort than the exact same procedure performed with the traditional scalpel technique.

For incisional carbon dioxide laser surgery, the tissue harvested with the focused laser beam can be examined histologically without difficulty since there is minimal thermal change caused by this laser. Also, for excisional laser surgery, undermining with the carbon dioxide laser in its focused mode of operation is extremely fast and simple. Yet, the surgeon can perform even complicated closures with full confidence that postoperative hematoma or seroma formation will be less likely to occur than with standard blunt or scalpel techniques.

In virtually all cases, the same type of closure technique utilized for conventional sharp excisional surgery can be used with laser surgical procedures as well. In spite of this, there is strong evidence that carbon dioxide laser incisions do not achieve the same tensile strength as scalpel-incised incisions until three weeks postoperatively. Thereafter, both types of wounds are indistinguishable from one another in cosmetic appearance and tensile strength. While the validity of this research is not questioned, this delay in development of tensile strength has not played a clinically significant role in the management of laser surgical wounds. It is possible that because of the quality of hemostasis achieved using the carbon dioxide laser for incisional surgery, the initial fibrin clot that usually forms after any kind of injury may not develop with the laser surgical technique. As a consequence, this may delay the initiation of fibroblast migration across the wound and the subsequent collagen synthesis and development of tensile strength. In any event, the laser surgeon performing carbon dioxide laser incision should recognize that this delay in tensile strength exists and should take whatever necessary precautions are required.

DISADVANTAGES OF CARBON DIOXIDE LASER SURGERY

Laser surgical procedures cannot be performed even by surgeons of great surgical skill with the same degree of precision or speed the first few times this instrumentation is utilized. Since the laser beam is the only portion of the laser instrument that contacts tissue, the surgeon may lose the normal tactile sensation of the scalpel blade contacting skin. When first beginning laser surgery, a small stylus may be used at the tip of the handpiece (Figure 128) in order to keep the laser beam precisely at its focal point. However, as one develops greater facility with the carbon dioxide laser, the stylus becomes an impediment and keeps the laser beam from being advanced into the open wound so that it is constantly kept in focus as the incision proceeds. Thus, some additional manual dexterity is required by the laser surgeon, at least in the beginning, before the carbon dioxide laser can be used with the same degree of skill previously obtained with traditional scalpel surgery. Also, the bulky nature and

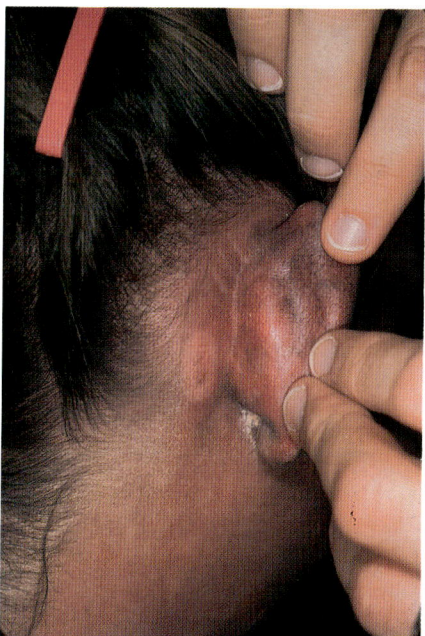

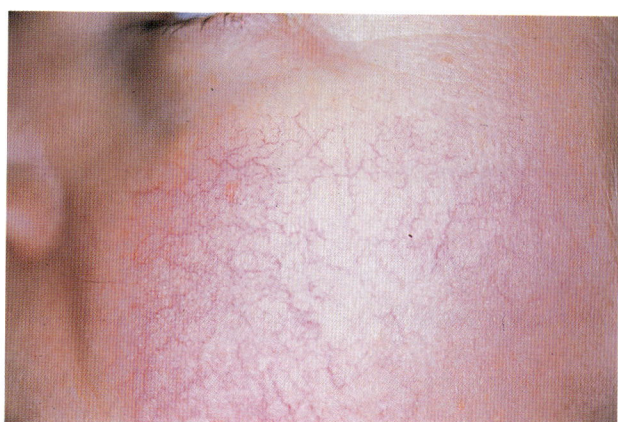

Figure 77.

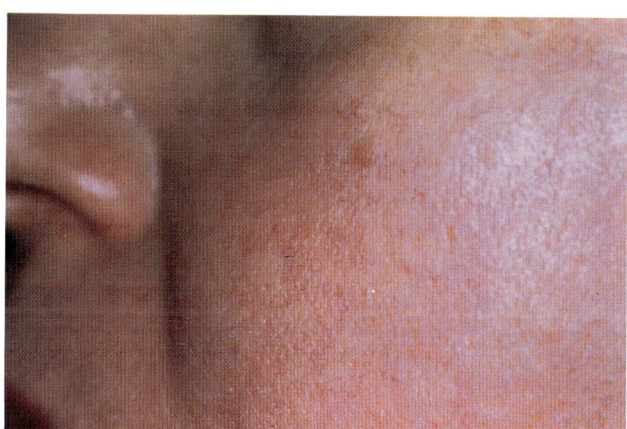

Figure 19.

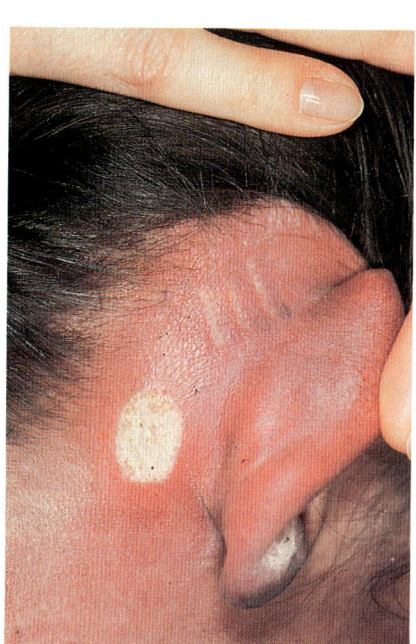

Figure 79.

Figure 81.

Figure 19. Same patient as in Figure 17, three months postoperatively, showing early lightening of four of the argon test sites and some lightening of the carbon dioxide laser test site.

Figure 77. Multiple telangiectatic blood vessels are seen on the cheek.

Figure 79. Final appearance six weeks after argon laser treatment of patient shown in Figure 77.

Figure 81. Profound blush reaction of the cheek immediately after argon laser treatment.

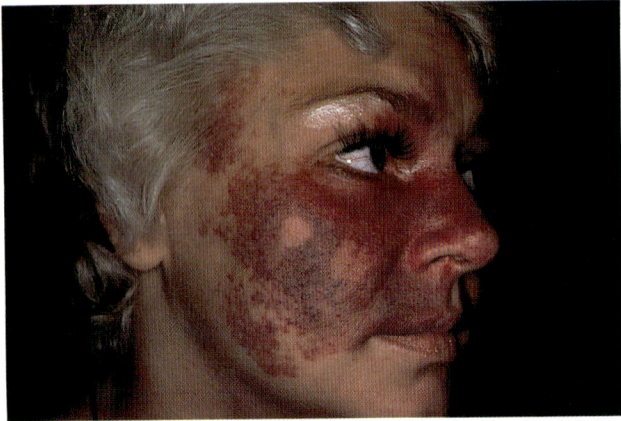

Figure 129.

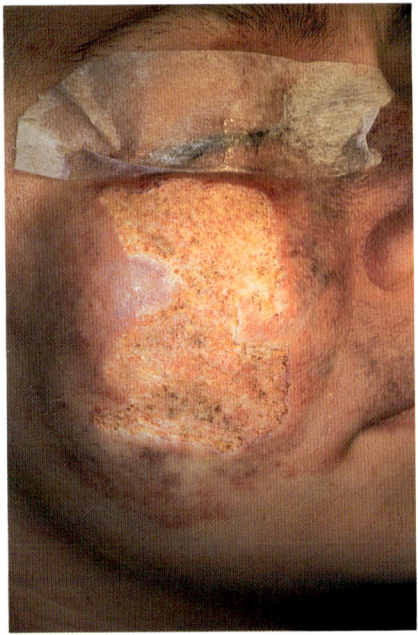

Figure 133.

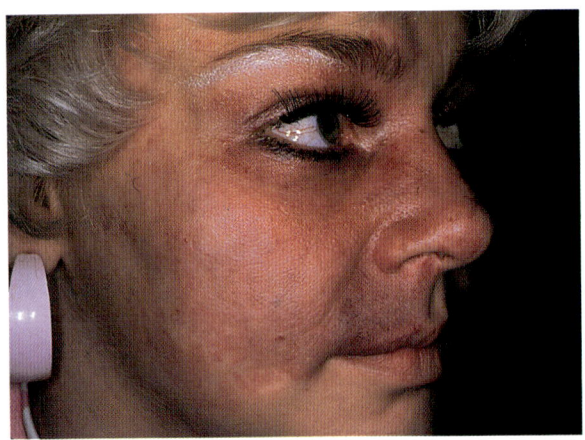

Figure 136.

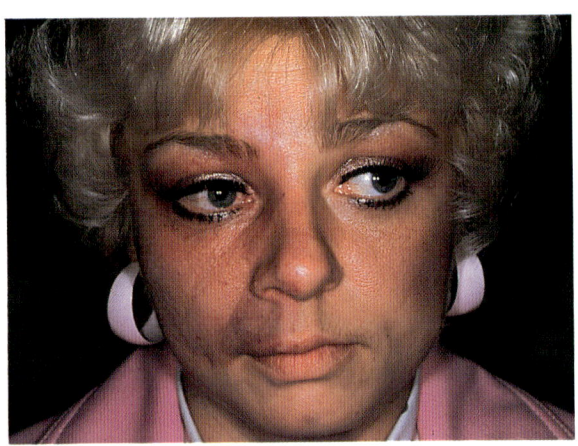

Figure 137.

Figure 129. Clinical appearance of a large portwine stain showing the lateral carbon dioxide laser test site and medial argon laser test sites three months after treatment.

Figure 133. Standard size of a carbon dioxide laser treatment site with blanching immediately post-laser treatment.

Figure 136. Appearance of the entire right cheek three months after laser treatment showing substantial improvement in color as well as texture of the nose and cheek.

Figure 137. Final appearance one year after laser treatment to the right cheek showing greater color on the affected side compared to the normal side, but still substantial improvement. [Note: Upper lip was not treated due to the potential increased risk of adverse scarring.]

4   Carbon Dioxide Laser Vaporization

When the carbon dioxide laser is used in its defocused mode, traditionally, the beam used is between 1 and 2 mm in diameter, the power setting on the instrument is 4 to 5 watts, resulting in an irradiance of between 130 to 640 watts/cm^2 (Table 6). When energy from the carbon dioxide laser beam strikes soft tissue, there is instantaneous conversion of cellular water into steam and smoke at 100°C. The precise control provided by this very shallow, 0.1 mm, zone of vaporization, allows accurate treatment of many skin conditions that are otherwise subject to scarring caused by treatment with imprecise, ablative nonlaser techniques.

ANGIOMA (PORTWINE STAIN)

The list of potential problems that can be treated with the carbon dioxide laser in its vaporizational mode is extremely long (Table 7). The techniques utilized in each of these conditions varies somewhat from one patient and one anatomic location to another, but there are many similarities in vaporizational treatment techniques. One vascular condition that has been successfully treated with the carbon dioxide laser is that of portwine stains. As previously discussed, the argon laser has been the traditional laser instrument used in the treatment of this condition. However, because the carbon dioxide laser can be used in a very precise fashion causing a very thin zone of destruction, the excess vascular tissue present in this type of angioma can be successfully removed using carbon dioxide laser vaporization. In this technique, a small representative portion of the portwine stain is vaporized as a test using 1% plain lidocaine anesthesia (Figure 129) (see color insert). When this is performed, the superficial dermal capillary plexus of ectatic vascular channels are instantaneously converted to steam and smoke and thermal sealing of the deeper blood vessels occurs. When the char on the surface is removed by cleansing with 3% hydrogen peroxide, persistent blood vessels that perforate vertically through the skin can be readily identified and subsequently vaporized with an immediate second treatment repetition. Usually, the size of the test

site is approximately 1 cm in diameter. In many laser centers, all angioma patients are tested using both the argon laser as well as the carbon dioxide laser. After testing, the patient is examined three to six months later to determine which laser produced the greatest improvement and to ensure that no adverse scarring has occurred.

After carbon dioxide laser treatment of a portwine stain, healing occurs by second intention. This requires much patient compliance during the two- to three-week interval necessary for this to occur. During this period, the patient must cleanse the wound twice daily with hydrogen peroxide followed by application of a fine film of Polysporin ointment and a small absorbant dressing on the surface. Once the wound has re-epithelialized, the treated portion of the angioma continues to appear red in color, but over a period of three to six months, permanent blanching begins. For angioma patients with a papular irregular surface, a substantial improvement in the textural irregularities can occur following treatment with the carbon dioxide laser.

At the follow-up visit, three to six months after performance of the carbon dioxide laser test on an angioma, the treatment site is carefully evaluated for evidence of improvement (Figure 129). This includes the percentage of lightening and the absence of scarring or other textural changes. If argon laser tests have also been performed, these are compared with the carbon dioxide test site. Whichever laser has given the greatest degree of improvement and provided the best cosmetic improvement is chosen to initiate therapy.

Generally, a treatment site of approximately 2 to 3 square inches is outlined on the patient's face and then photography is performed. Injection of 1% plain lidocaine is utilized for anesthesia since vasoconstriction is unnecessary for hemostasis. Then, with the laser set at 4 to 5 watts and using a 2 mm beam, one entire layer of the treatment site is superficially vaporized. The wound is then cleansed by light rubbing with hydrogen peroxide and any persistent vessels or perforating blood vessels that remain are treated in similar fashion. Usually only two or three layers are treated to completely remove all vessels (Figure 130). A sterile dressing is applied and the patient is given wound care instructions (Figures 131

Table 6. CO₂ Laser Vaporization

Power 4–5 watts
Irradiance* 130–640 watts/cm²
Pulsed or continuous mode
Defocused 1–2 mm impact spot size (beam diameter)
Penetration depth of 0.1 mm

Advantages
  Precise control
  No scatter or heat conduction
  Total energy absorption in 100 micra of water or living tissue
  Bloodless field to increase visibility
  Permits surgery in tight locations, eg. external auditory canal, inner canthi, perianal tissue
  Hemostasis—seals blood vessels up to 0.5 mm in diameter
  Lymphatics sealed to decrease postoperative swelling
  Decreased postoperative pain
  Works even in anticoagulated patients
  No effect on pacemakers
  Minimal damage to normal tissue

Disadvantages
  Expense of equipment
  Bulky handpiece
  Smoke and smell
  Safety precautions

$$* \text{ Irradiance} = \frac{\text{power (watts)}}{\pi \times \text{radius of beam (cm)}^2}$$

Table 7. Skin Conditions Treatable by the CO₂ Laser

Vaporization (defocused) mode of operation
  Proliferative disorders
    Warts—flat or common type
    Actinic cheilitis
    Trichoepithelioma
    Syringoma
    Adenoma Sebaceum
    Neurofibroma
    Epidermal nevi
    Xanthelasma
    Eruptive vellus hair cysts
    Seborrheic keratosis (large)
    Actinic keratoses (multiple)
    Rhinophyma
  Vascular conditions
    Portwine stain
    Senile (cherry) angioma
    Pyogenic granuloma
    Lymphangioma
  Miscellaneous conditions
    Laserabrasion of scars
    Decorative tattoo
    Traumatic tattoo

and 132). Postoperatively, there may be a minor burning sensation but discomfort rarely requires use of narcotic analgesics.

Treatment is continued with additional segments vaporized every five to six weeks until therapy is completed (Figures 133–135) (see color insert). Final lightening, as with the argon laser, does not occur until 12 to 18 months postoperatively for most patients. While the improvement in texture occurs very quickly, the final blanching is somewhat delayed (Figures 136 and 137) (see color insert). If portions of the angioma have failed to clear substantially or if a few small ectatic vessels remain, these areas can be revaporized after this time interval has passed.

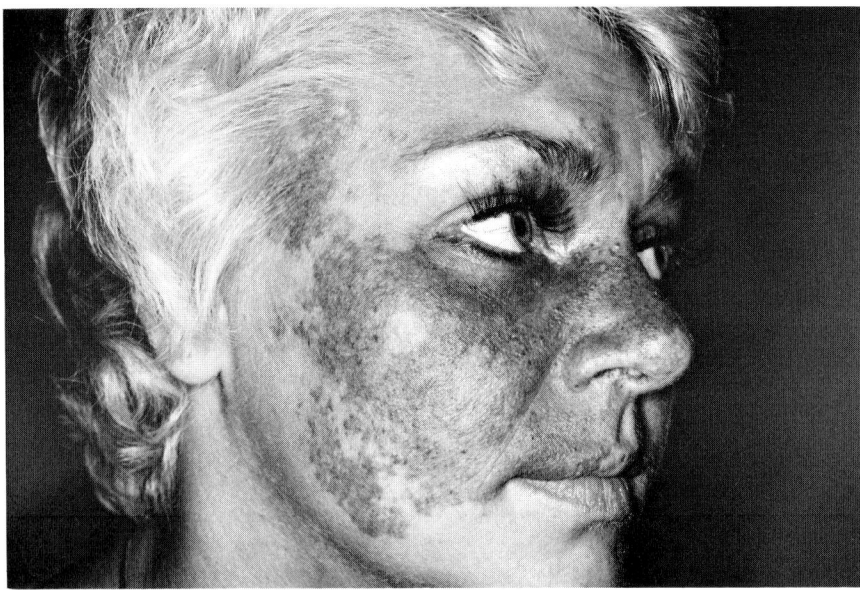

Figure 129. Clinical appearance of a large portwine stain showing the lateral carbon dioxide laser test site and medial argon laser test sites three months after treatment.

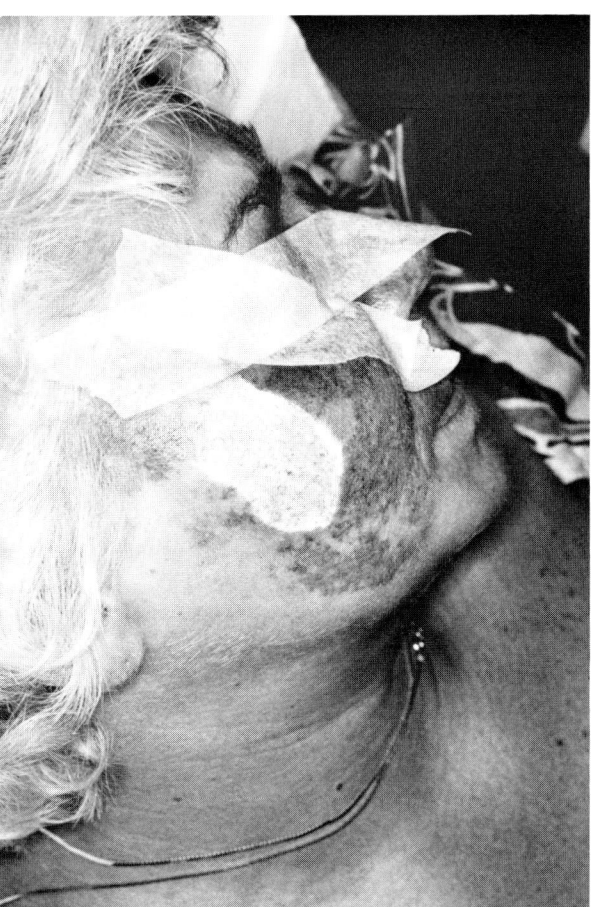

Figure 130. Appearance of patient seen in Figure 129 immediately after a small segment of the portwine stain has been vaporized using the carbon dioxide laser. The base appears somewhat lighter in color than the surrounding skin due to the bleaching effects of hydrogen peroxide.

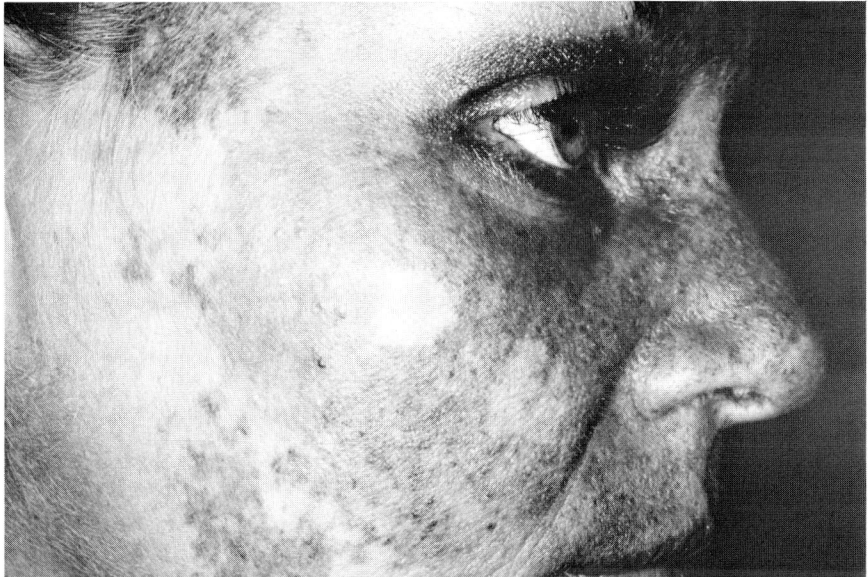

Figure 131. Same patient identified in Figure 129 six weeks postoperatively showing substantial improvement in the angiomatous color.

Figure 132. Same patient seen in Figure 129 three months after carbon dioxide laser treatment of the right lateral superior cheek segment showing additional lightening in color.

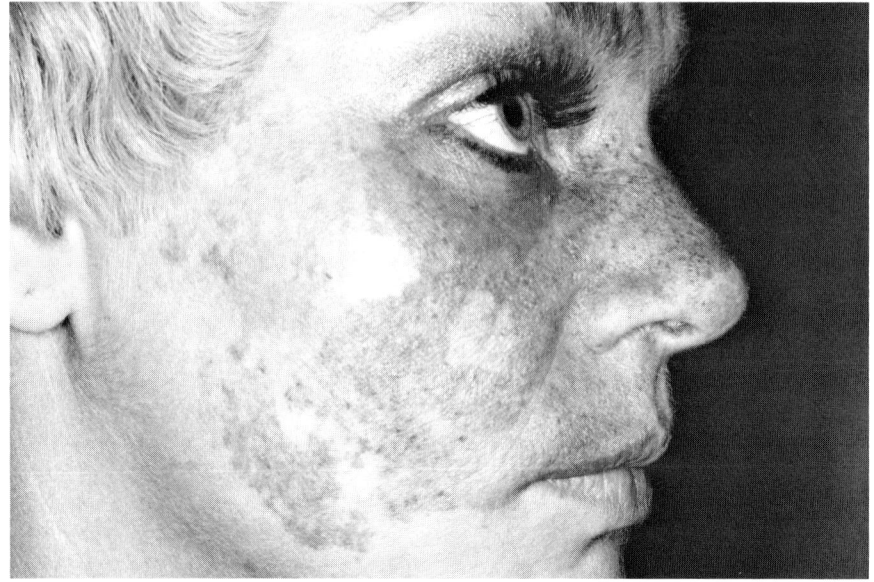

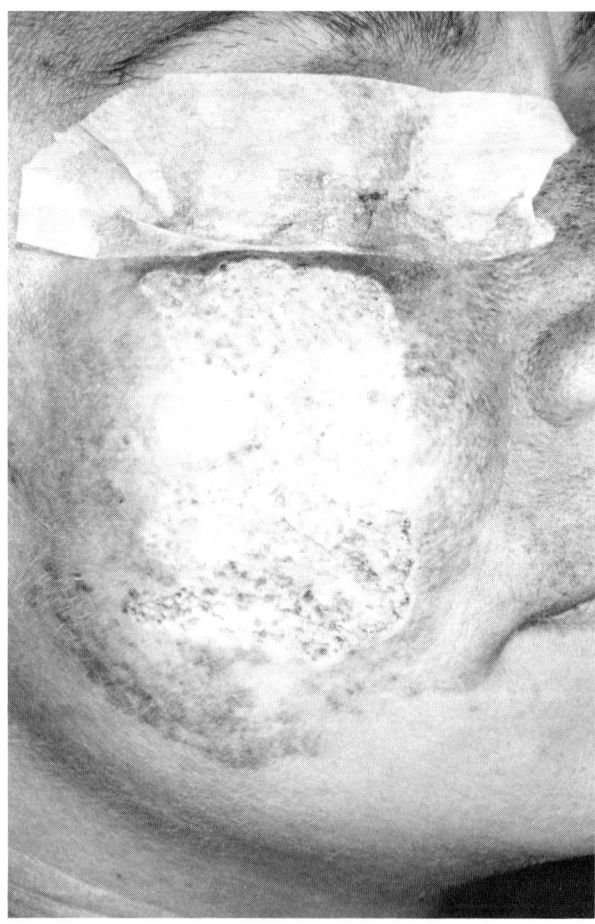

Figure 133. Standard size of a carbon dioxide laser treatment site with blanching immediately post-laser treatment.

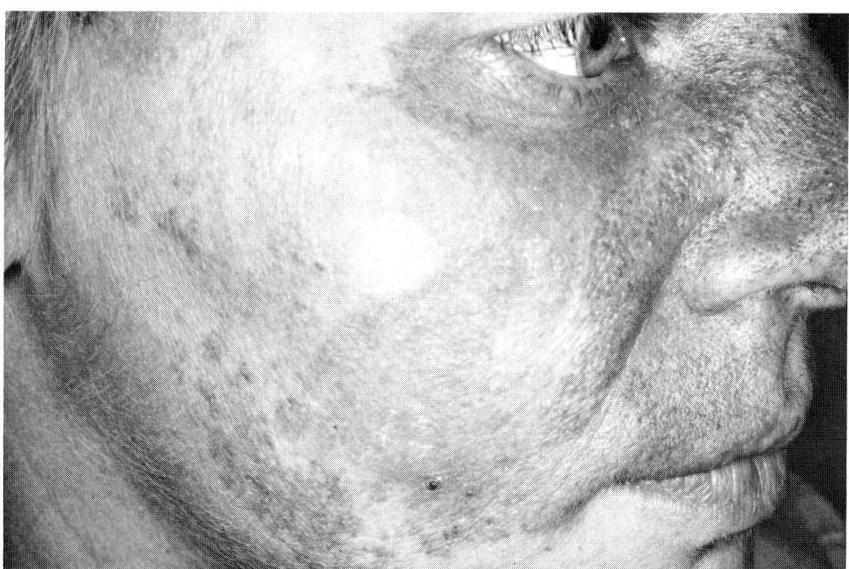

Figure 134. Residual erythema and some postinflammatory hyperpigmentation is seen in the treatment site demonstrated in Figure 133 one month post-laser treatment.

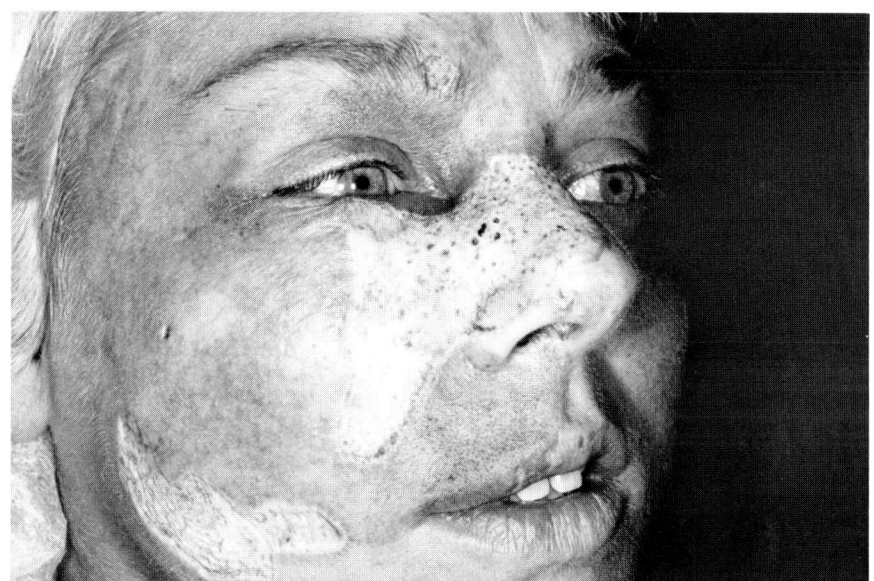

Figure 135. Two segments have been treated on this patient using the carbon dioxide laser on the nose, medial cheek and jawline. No bleeding is present. (See Figures 136 and 137.)

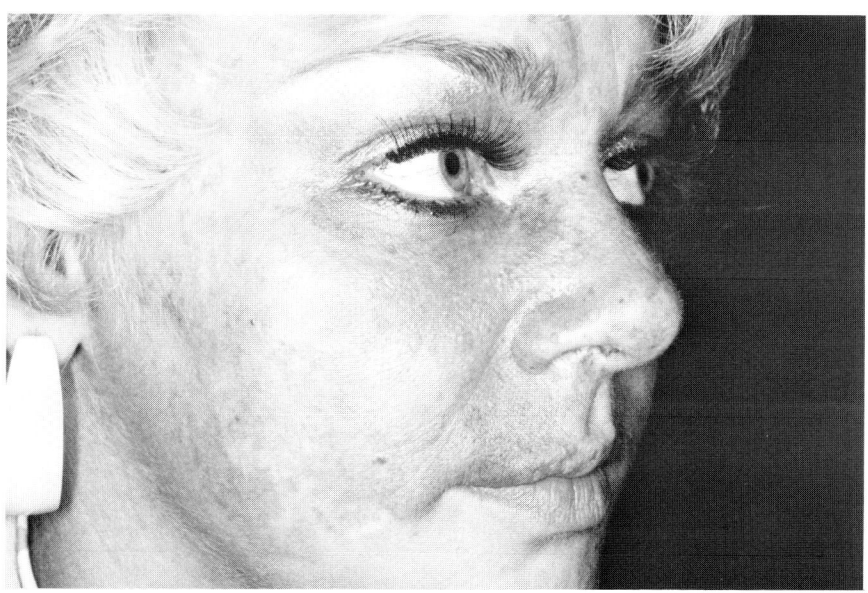

Figure 136. Appearance of the entire right cheek of patient identified in Figure 135 three months after laser treatment showing substantial improvement in color as well as texture.

Figure 137. Final appearance (same patient as in Figure 135) one year after laser treatment to the right cheek showing greater color on the affected side compared to the normal side, but still substantial improvement.

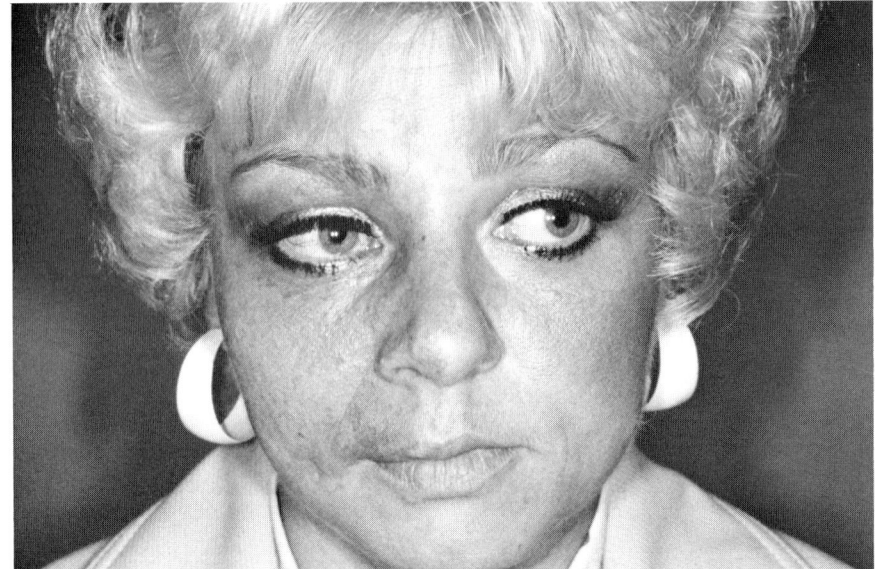

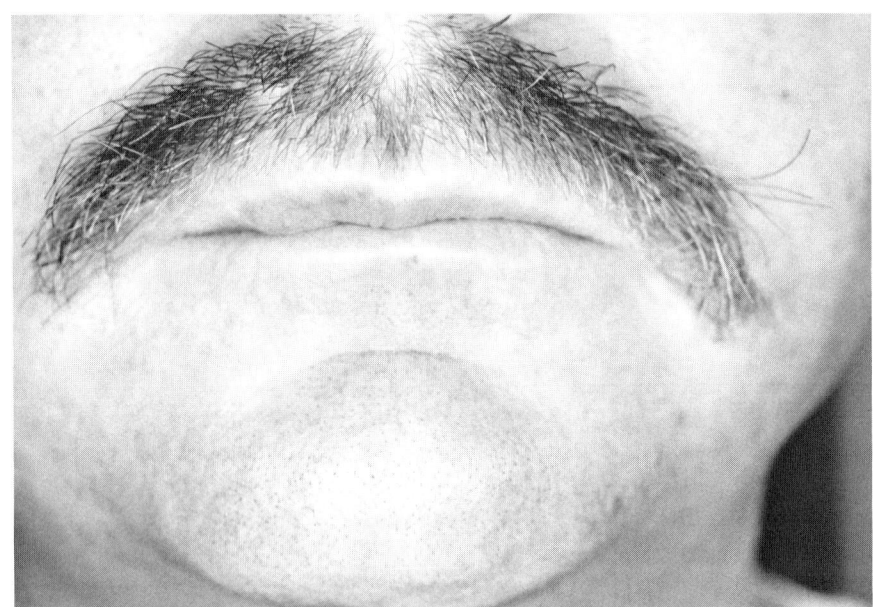

Figure 138. Numerous small, bluish-black, traumatic tattoos of the chin and lower lip preoperatively.

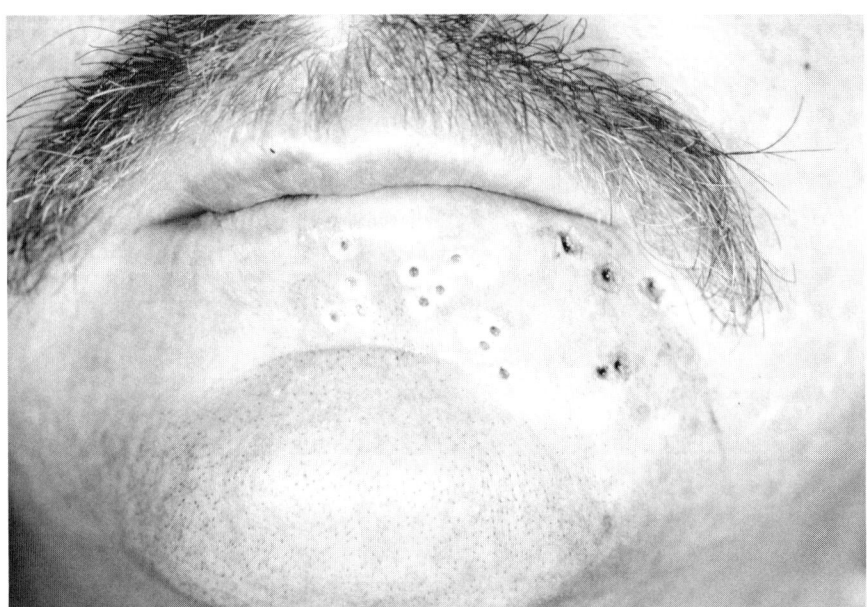

Figure 139. Small areas have been vaporized from the affected site until all pigment has been removed. (Same patient as seen in Figure 138.)

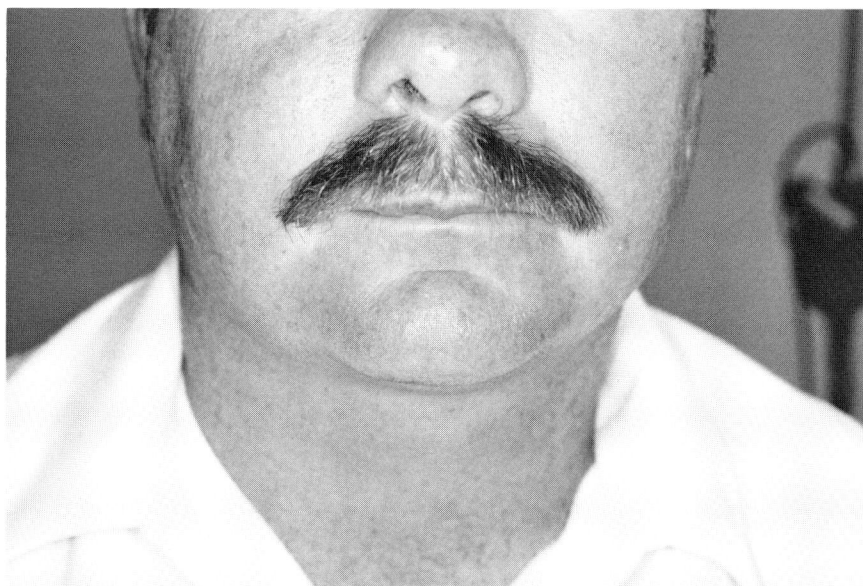

Figure 140. Clinical appearance showing no residual pigmentation three months postoperatively and an excellent cosmetic result for patient seen in Figure 138.

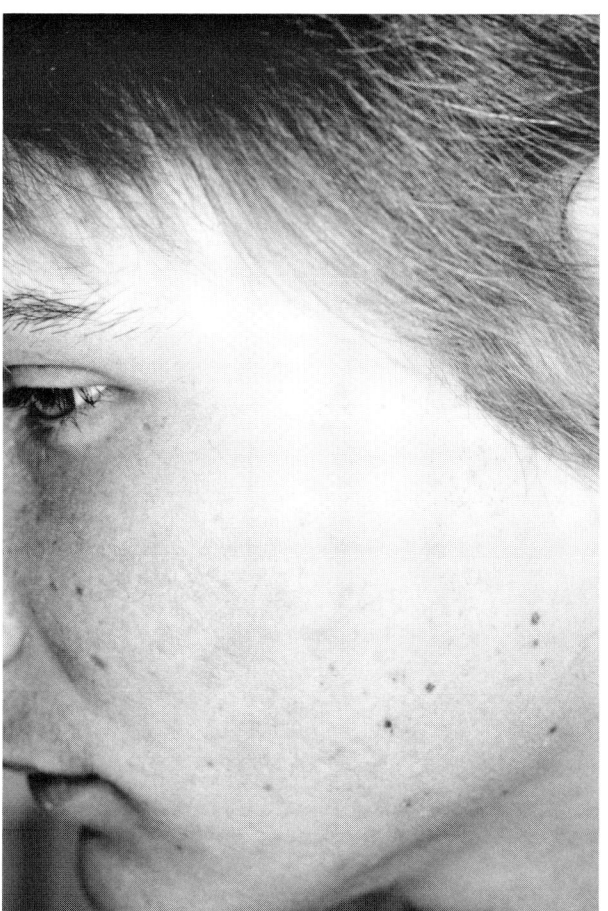

Figure 141. Numerous small, bluish-black, traumatic tattoos of the left cheek preoperatively. (See Figures 142 and 143.)

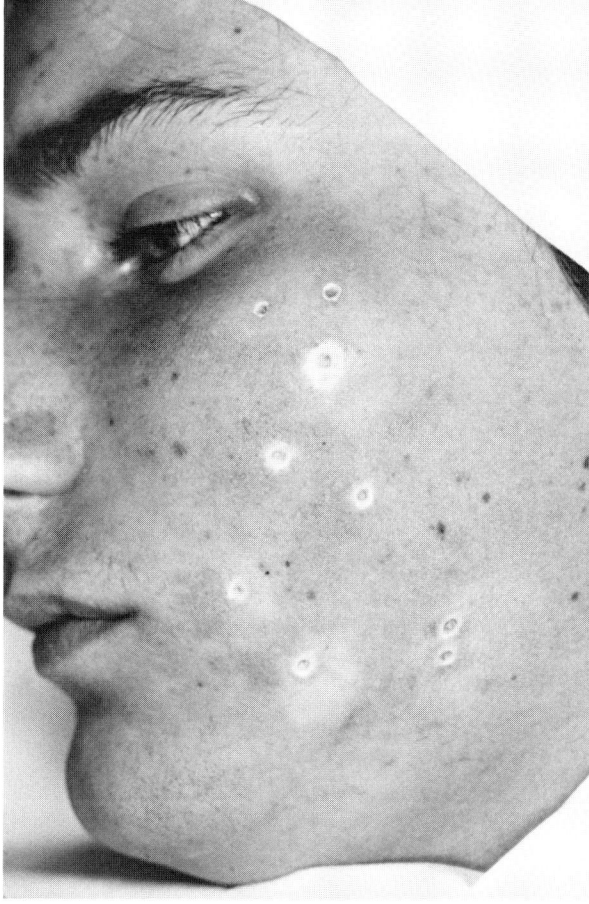

Figure 142. Superficial vaporization of the affected zones has removed all pigment.

Figure 143. Residual postinflammatory, hyperpigmentation and some textural scarring is evident six weeks post-laser treatment.

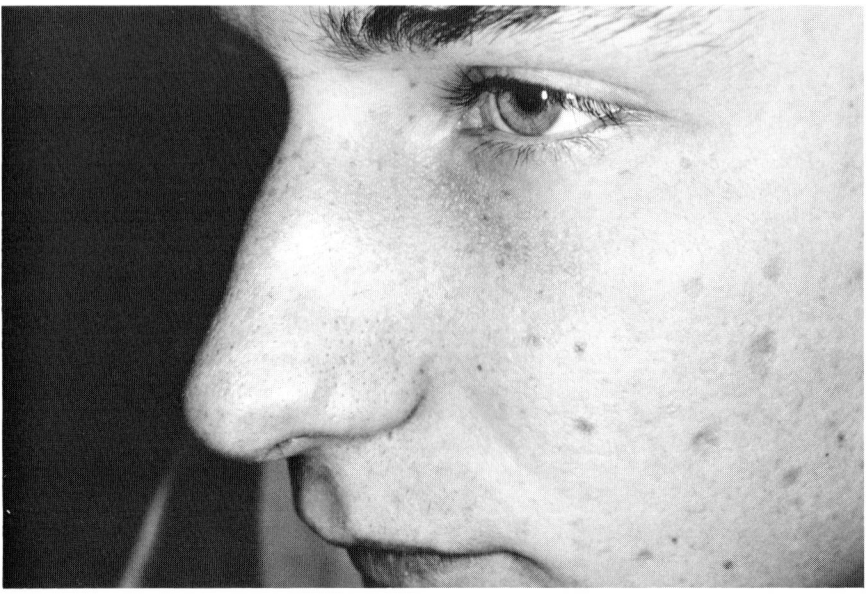

TATTOOS

Fortunately, decorative tattoos are not commonly found on the face. However, traumatic tattoos are a common occurrence in this area. The carbon dioxide laser can be used in the treatment of both of these conditions in a very satisfactory fashion. Again, if large areas are affected, treatment of a small representative test site is preferable for decorative tattoos. However, there may be a disadvantage in delaying treatment of traumatic tattoos since phagocytic cells may engulf the foreign pigment soon after injury and move it deeper into the tissue and make subsequent removal more difficult. As a consequence, many laser surgeons will treat the entire zone of traumatic tattooing on the head and neck in a single session to minimize the chances of deeper absorption of pigment and further disfigurement, accepting the potential risk of adverse scarring or irregular texture after healing as unavoidable.

For the treatment of tattoos of the head and neck, local anesthesia is required. However, for

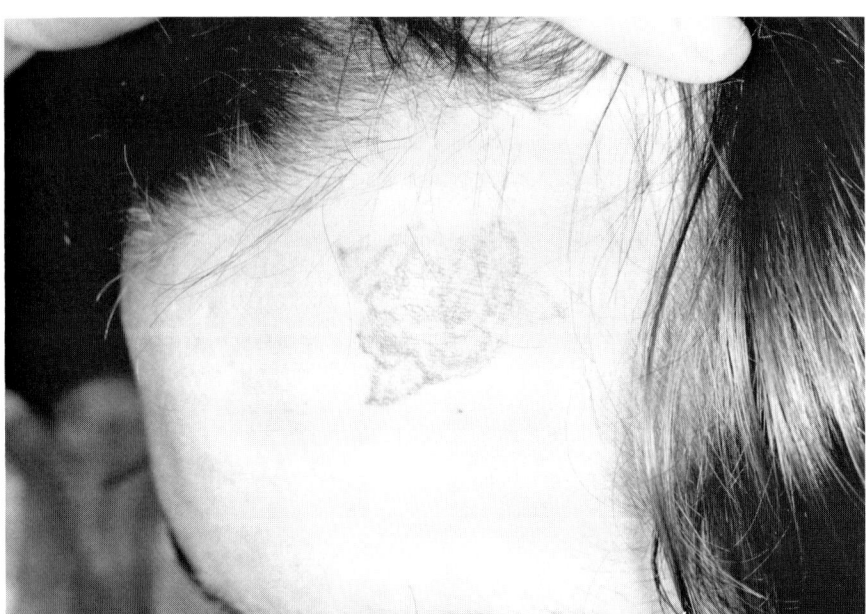

Figure 144. Decorative tattoo of the forehead preoperatively. (See Figures 145–147.)

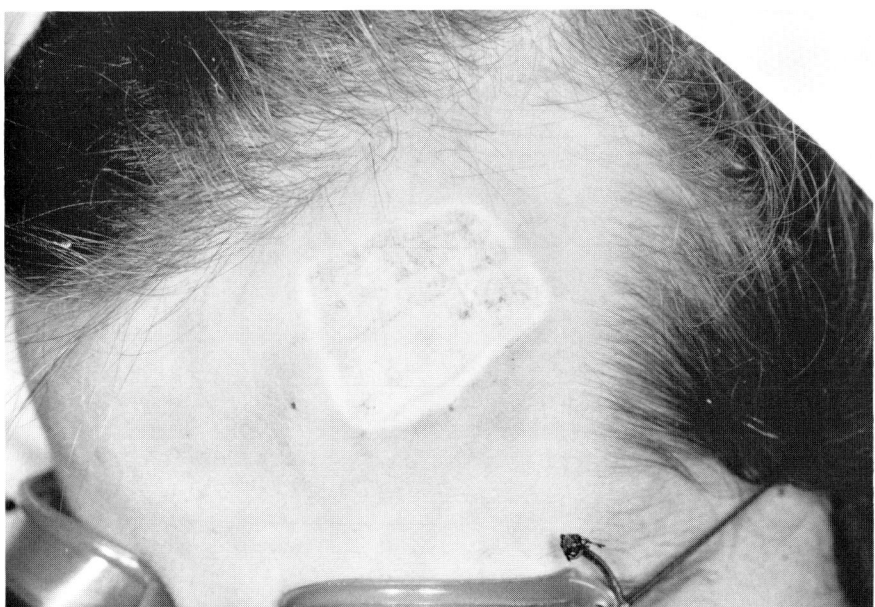

Figure 145. Vaporization has been performed of the entire tattoo and a small amount of normal skin to create a different shape or design.

large decorative tattoos, circumferential injections of 1% lidocaine with epinephrine 1 : 200,000 is utilized. If larger areas of the face are to be treated as with traumatic tattoos from powder explosions (Figures 138–143), nerve block anesthesia or general anesthesia may be required. The laser is set at a power setting of 4 to 5 watts and a 2 mm defocused laser beam is utilized. In this case, the carbon dioxide laser may be set to deliver brief pulses of laser energy of between 0.1 and 0.5 seconds in duration. With this pulsed technique, the small zones of trau-

matic tattoo pigment can be individually vaporized followed by cleansing after each pass to ensure adequacy of removal.

For larger professional decorative facial tattoos (Figures 144–147), the carbon dioxide laser is typically employed with similar laser parameters, but in a continuous discharge mode. Between each pass, the surface char and debris are removed with light scrubbing using a cotton gauze 2 × 2 or cotton-tipped applicators soaked in 3% hydrogen peroxide. If residual tattoo pigment remains, it is selectively vaporized

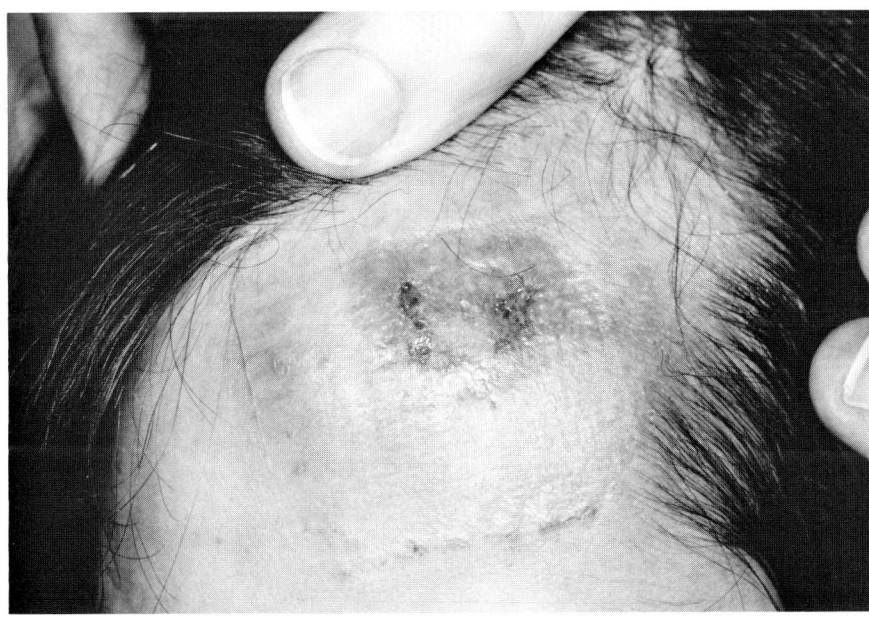

Figure 146. Same patient identified in Figure 144. Healing of the treatment site four weeks postoperatively.

Figure 147. Appearance of treatmet site four months postoperatively showing textural change and some slight residual erythema.

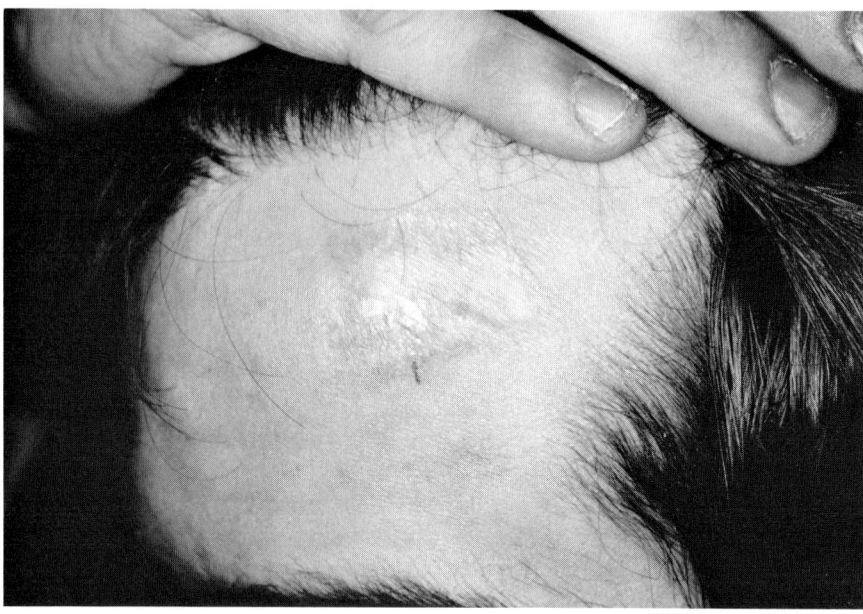

layer by layer until all pigment has been completely removed. This removal process can frequently be more carefully performed with use of 2.5 x magnification loupes. It must be remembered that if a decorative tattoo has a distinctive shape or name, the sharp margins must be contoured so that the healed scar will not duplicate the original appearance of the tattoo and be equally offensive to the patient.

Once laser treatment has been completed, all char is removed again with 3% hydrogen peroxide scrubbing and a small amount of antibacterial ointment is applied. A small sterile dressing is put on the surface and the patient is instructed to cleanse the wound with 3% hydrogen peroxide twice daily followed by application of a thin film of antibiotic ointment. The treatment site heals by second intention over a period of three to four weeks depending on the anatomic location, depth of original tattoo pigmentation, and diligence of wound care by the individual patient. At first, the wound may appear much darker or redder than the surrounding normal tissue, but with time the pigmentary changes at the treatment site will resolve and with careful sunlight restriction, satisfactory cosmetic results can be obtained in most patients within 12 to 18 months.

The main advantage of using the carbon dioxide laser in its vaporizational mode of operation over that of dermabrasion or salabrasion for the treatment of tattoos is virtually complete pigment removal in one operative procedure. The excellent visual control provided by using the carbon dioxide laser in this mode of operation

ensures complete pigment removal. Also, most patients will have less postoperative discomfort when carbon dioxide laser vaporization is used compared to the more traditional tattoo removal techniques.

All patients who undergo laser treatment for tattoos of the head and neck must recognize that with tattoo removal there will be some permanent textural change or scarring. Many patients have the ill-conceived notion that laser surgery can effectively remove lesions of this type without any cosmetic deformity. Sadly, this misconception must be fully explained at the initial consultative visit to prevent unhappy consequences after completion of this procedure.

LASER VAPORIZATION OF ACTINIC CHEILITIS

One condition where significant advantages are offered by the carbon dioxide laser is in the treatment of severely sun-damaged lips known as actinic cheilitis (Figure 148). Previous treatment was, at best, poor and subject to numerous complications as well as significant cosmetic deformity. For the laser technique, the lower lip is made anesthetic either through nerve block or local infiltration of 1% lidocaine with epinephrine 1 : 200,000. The laser is set at 4 to 6 watts of power and a 2 mm beam diameter is used to deliver defocused carbon dioxide laser energy to the affected tissue, which has first been outlined

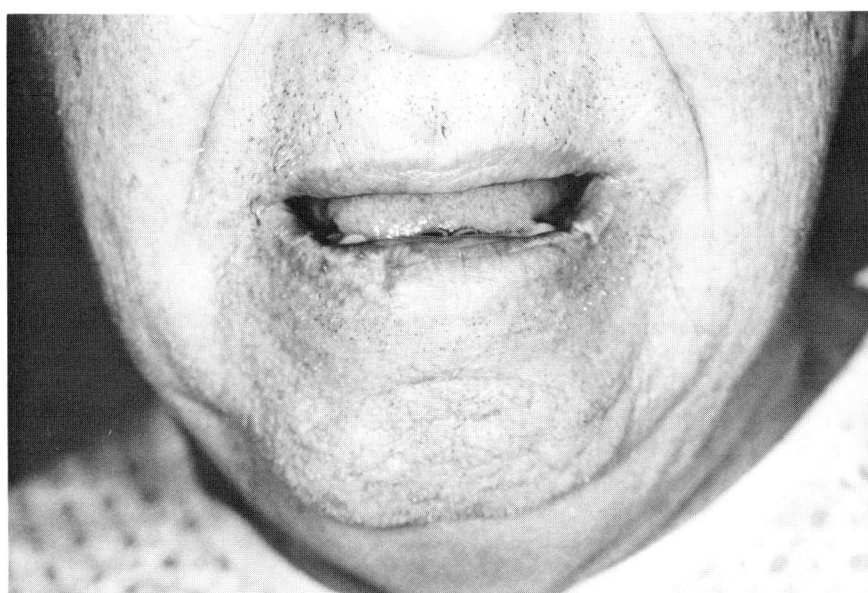

Figure 148. Severe actinic cheilitis of the lower lip preoperatively. (See Figures 149–151.)

with surgical marking ink. One entire layer is vaporized in this fashion and the surface char is then removed with 3% hydrogen peroxide (Figure 149). Areas of persistent abnormal epithelium are bleached by the hydrogen peroxide and typically have a slightly whiter color than the normal surrounding tissue. These persistent zones of involvement are revaporized using similar settings. After all abnormal tissue has been removed, the wound is dressed with application of an antibiotic ointment, absorbant gauze, and held in place with paper tape.

The main advantage of this technique is that postoperatively, patients have very little discomfort and can function without difficulty in most situations (Figure 150). They are able to eat and drink in the usual fashion without much difficulty. Over a period of 12 to 14 days, the wound heals by second intention and the final cosmetic results in most cases are superb with excellent color and texture (Figure 151). The limited zone of destruction caused by the precise delivery of carbon dioxide laser energy is responsible for this excellent result.

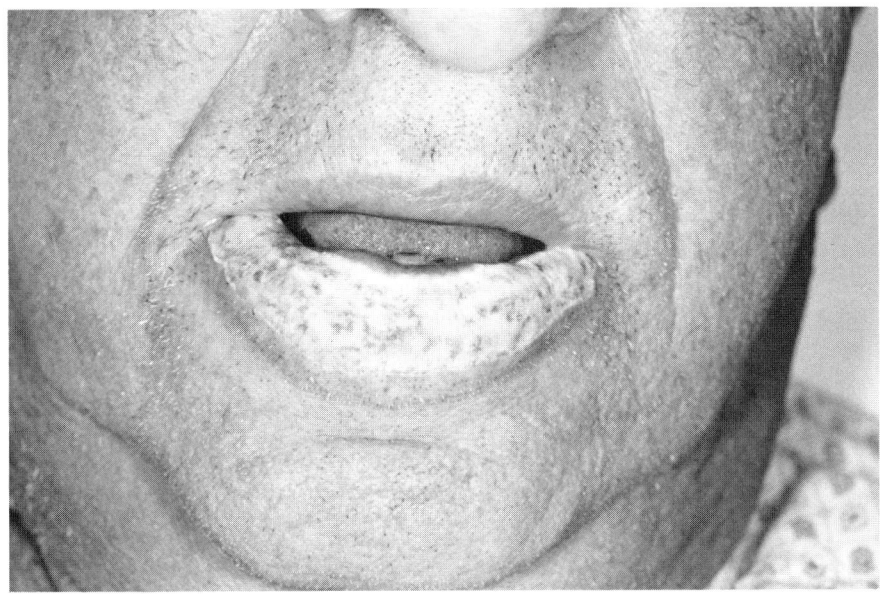

Figure 149. One entire layer of the lower lip has been vaporized using the carbon dioxide laser and the char removed with hydrogen peroxide which accounts for the white discoloration.

Figure 150. Superficial crusting and minimal edema is seen five days post-laser treatment.

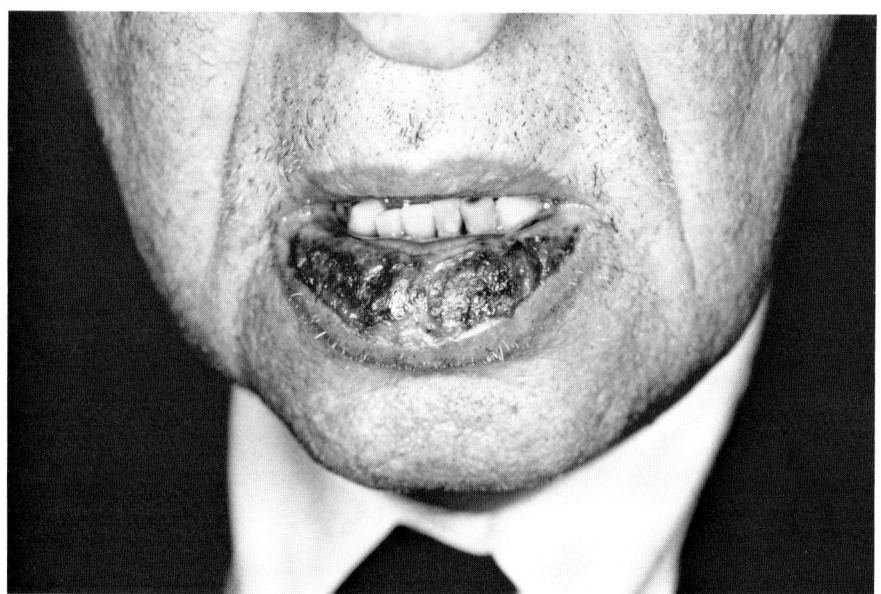

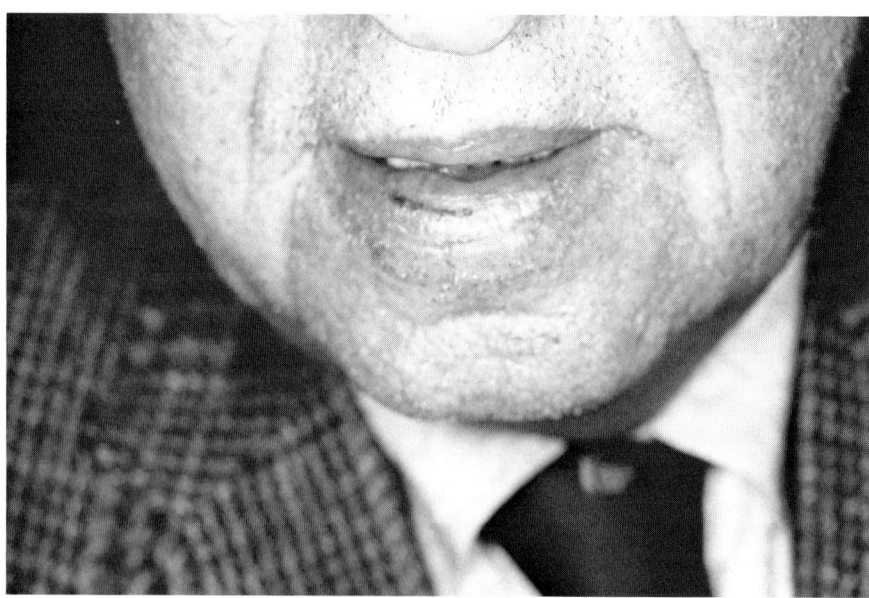

Figure 151. Complete healing with excellent cosmetic results are evidenced by four weeks postoperatively.

MISCELLANEOUS CUTANEOUS LESIONS TREATED WITH CARBON DIOXIDE LASER VAPORIZATION

A number of appendageal tumors can be treated successfully with the carbon dioxide laser where prior therapy was either likely to result in scarring or have an otherwise unsatisfactory result. Several of these conditions that lend themselves quite readily to carbon dioxide laser vaporization are: syringoma, trichoepithelioma, adenoma sebaceum, and vellus hair cysts. In addition, the inflammatory condition known as granulom faciale, the vascular proliferation of pyogenic granuloma, and xanthelasma can also be treated in a similar fashion. Each of these will be discussed separately.

Syringoma

Each syringoma represents a collection of eccrine sweat glands and ducts and appears clinically as a small flesh-colored 1 to 3 mm papule that has a dome-shaped, smooth surface. These multiple lesions are found on the face and typically occur in the periorbital areas, but may also be found on the cheeks and forehead (Figure 152). These benign lesions can be treated with a variety of techniques but the laser can permit precise removal of the proliferating tissue with minimal injury to surrounding skin and an excellent cosmetic result.

The technique utilized for treatment of syringomas includes first marking each individual lesion with a surgical marking device. Local anesthesia is then obtained through intradermal injection of 1% lidocaine with epinephrine 1 : 200,000. The normal safety prcautions are utilized, since these lesions are found around the eyes, and either wet gauzes or small plastic goggles are placed over the patient's eyes to protect them against inadvertent damage by the laser. The laser is set at 4 watts of power and a defocused beam of 2 mm in diameter is used to deliver 0.10 seconds or 0.20 second pulses of energy to each individual lesion.

Usually only two or three pulses are required to completely remove each lesion. After treatment is complete, the individual sites of vaporization are cleansed with hydrogen peroxide and the base of each wound is carefully examined for the presence of additional syringoma tissue. This is usually identified as whitish-yellow material having a different texture than that of the surrounding normal tissue. If residual syringoma is identified, a second treatment pass is performed to the areas that persist (Figure 153). This procedure is repeated until all lesions have been treated. The wound is then dressed in the standard fashion and complete healing usually occurs within 12 to 14 days (Figure 154).

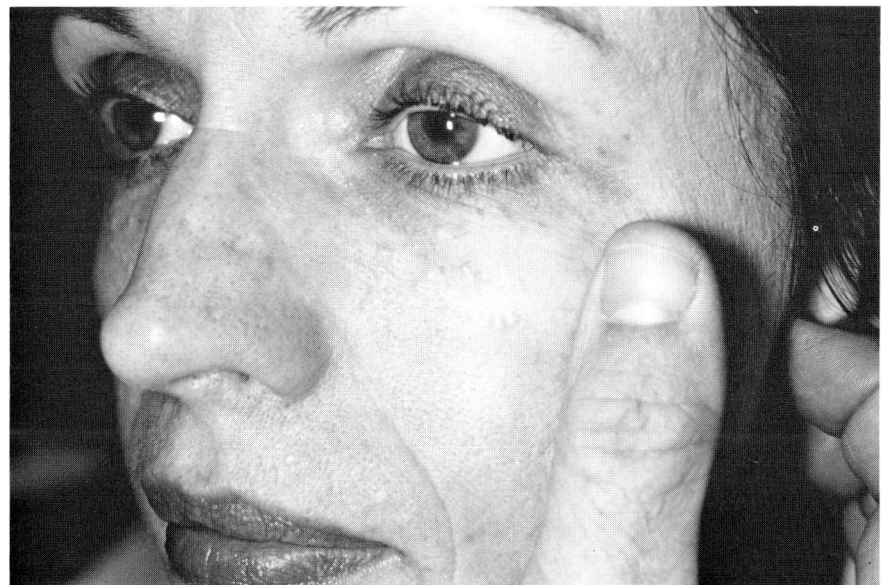

Figure 152. Numerous, small syringomas are identified on the left medial cheek preoperatively.

Figure 153. Same patient seen in Figure 152. After superficial vaporization using the carbon dioxide laser, small superficial wounds have been created.

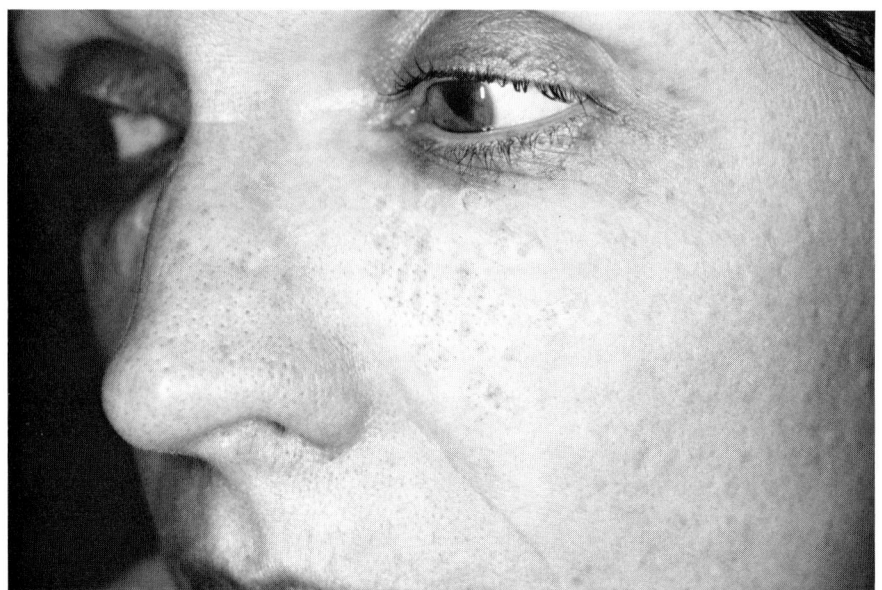

Figure 154. The final cosmetic results present at six weeks post-operatively showing no recurrent syringomatous growth and no adverse scarring or textural change noted. (Same patient seen in Figure 152.)

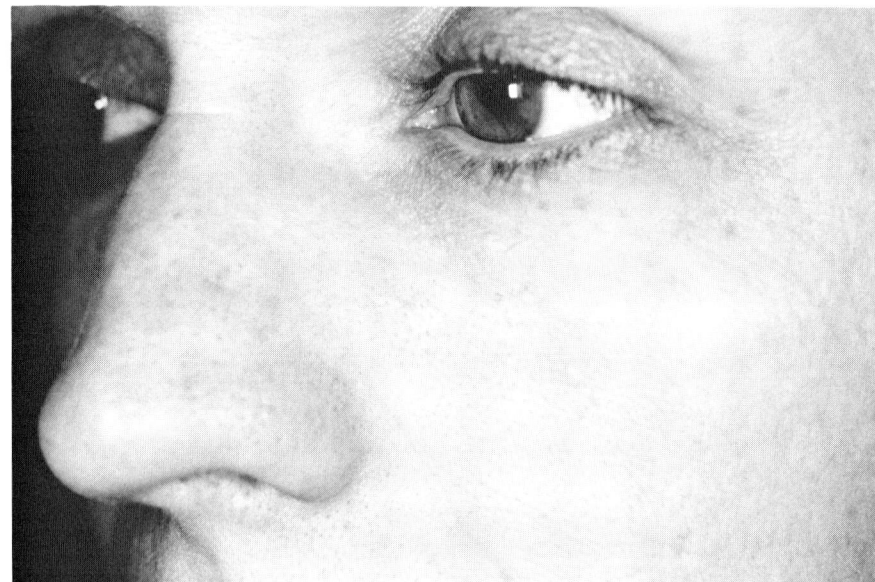

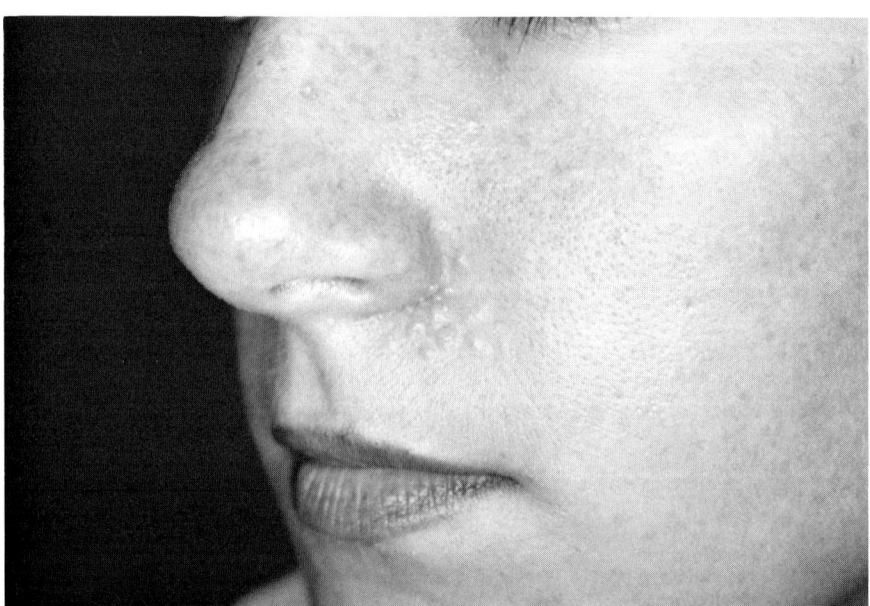

Figure 155. Translucent 3 mm papules of trichoepithelioma are noted adjacent to the nasolabial fold.

Trichoepithelioma

These benign hair-follicle tumors tend to occur most commonly in the perinasal and central facial areas as multiple, 3 to 8 mm, red or flesh-colored, slightly translucent, dome-shaped papules (Figure 155). The carbon dioxide laser is used to treat these lesions in a fashion similar to that described for syringomas with treatment under local anesthesia. The laser is again set at 4 to 6 watts of power and using a 2 mm beam, brief 0.10 seconds to 0.20 seconds pulses of laser energy are delivered to the surface of each individual papule which has been marked with surgical ink (Figure 156). Each lesion is treated until it is flat with the surrounding skin and then the surface char is removed with 3% hydrogen peroxide and the base of each wound is examined for possible remnants of trichoepithelioma. If these are present, additional passes are repeated until this tissue is completely removed (Figure 157). Stan-

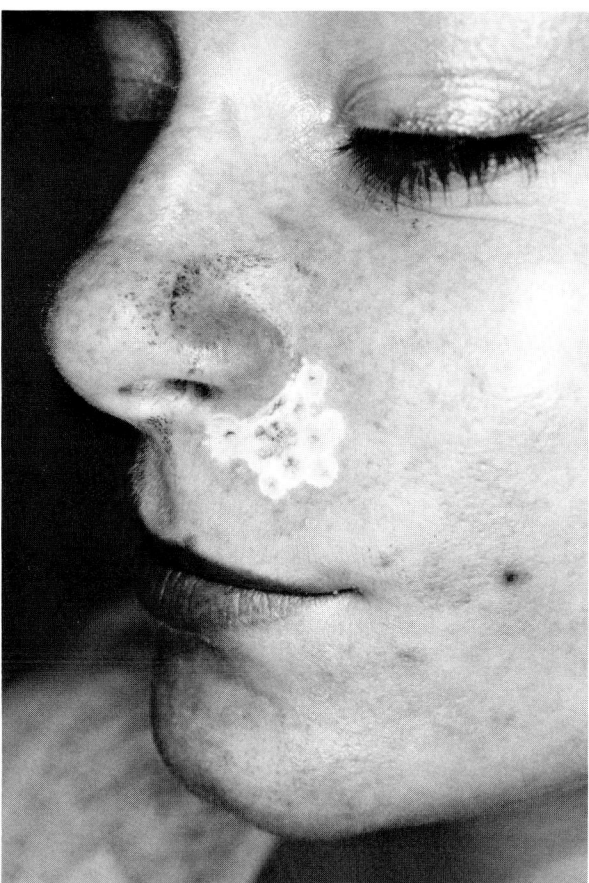

Figure 157. Appearance of patient shown in Figure 155 immediately postoperatively showing superficial defects caused by carbon dioxide laser vaporization.

dard dressings are employed and wound healing occurs in most cases uneventfully in 2 to 3 weeks (Figure 158).

Adenoma Sebaceum

These clinical lesions are sometimes seen in the syndrome of tuberous sclerosis and may be associated with mental retardation and seizures. However, there are individuals with this syndrome who only develop the soft tissue abnormality known as adenoma sebaceum. These papules represent proliferations of fibrovascular structures and do not relate, as their name would imply, to the pilosebaceous structure. These lesions typically occur on the central face and because they are usually present in great numbers, may be very disfiguring (Figure 159). The treatment for this difficulty is more generalized than that described above for both syringoma and trichoepithelioma since the zone of involvement is much greater.

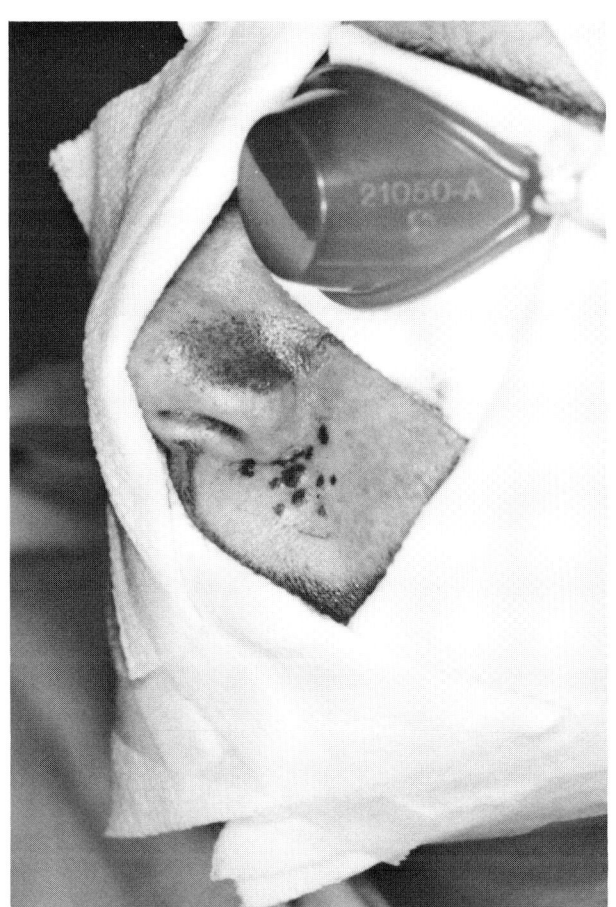

Figure 156. Same patient identified in Figure 155. The areas to be treated have been marked with surgical ink, eyes have been protected, and wet surgical drapes have been placed around the operative site for safety purposes.

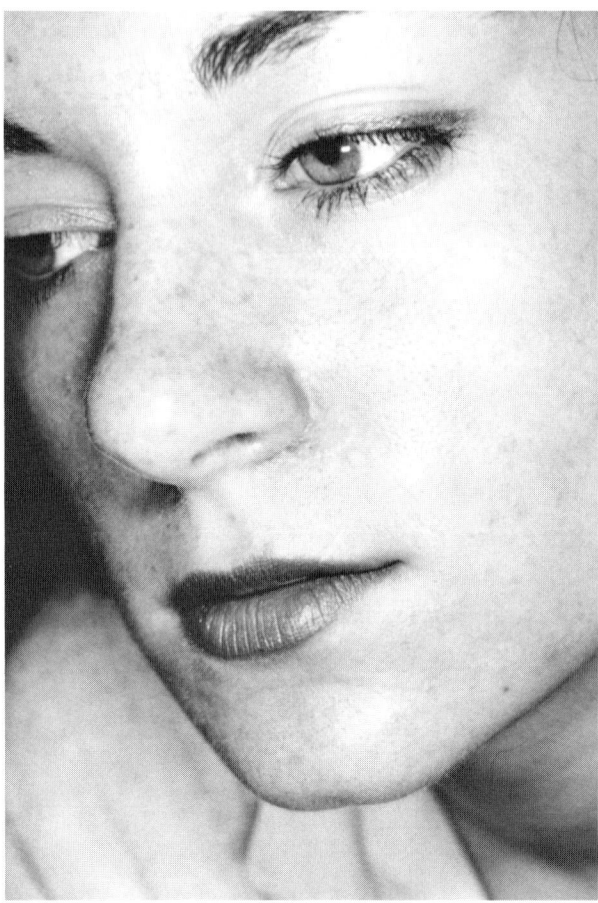

Figure 158. Same patient shown in Figure 155 six weeks postoperatively showing excellent cosmetic result without textural change or evidence of regrowth of trichoepithelioma.

pain postoperatively. Wound healing is similar to that which is seen for the dermabraded wound (Figures 161 and 162). Regrowth of these lesions can occur if the depth of each lesion is not adequately treated. However, a compromise must be reached in some patients where the depth of involvement required for total ablation would create an otherwise unsatisfactory scar. In these cases, retreatment may be performed on any areas that redevelop after the initial laser treatment.

Vellus Hair Cyst

These rather uncommon inherited lesions represent small collections of pilosebaceous structures typically distributed on the central face and periorbital areas. These well encapsulated cystic structures may be the cause of much disfigurement due to their cobblestone-type of appearance (Figure 163). This type of lesion can be

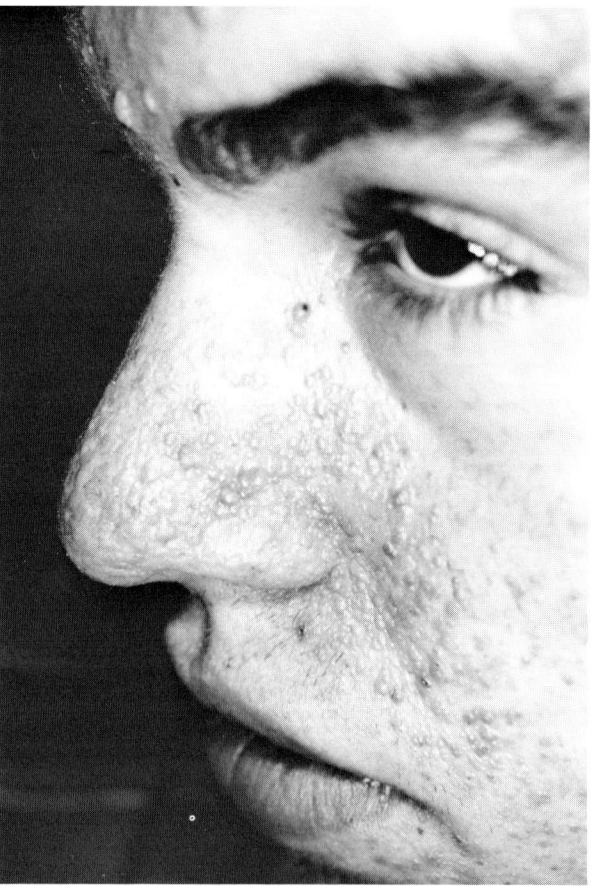

Figure 159. Preoperative appearance of a patient with adenoma sebaceum of the central face. (See Figures 160–162.)

In this situation, using either local anesthesia or nerve block, the affected area is anesthetized and the treatment zone is outlined with a surgical marker. The laser is set at 4 to 6 watts of power and with a 2 mm beam, carbon dioxide laser energy is continuously delivered to the entire affected zone of involvement (Figure 160). This has been called laserabrasion or lasabrasion when, in fact, neither is exactly true. What occurs during this treatment process is the superficial layers of the skin including the abnormal adenoma sebaceum lesions are vaporized. After one layer of the entire zone of involvement has been vaporized, the area is cleansed with hydrogen peroxide and the base of the wound is examined for persistent areas of involvement. These focal areas are subsequently treated with second or third repetitions of the above technique as necessary. The final defect is similar to that created with dermabrasion, but there is usually minimal

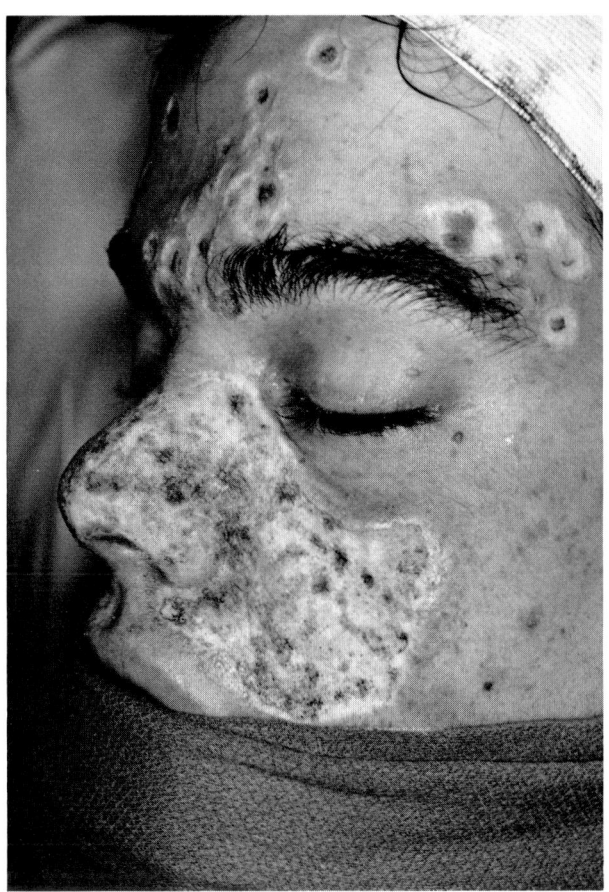

Figure 160. Same patient seen in Figure 159 immediately after carbon dioxide laser vaporization of the entire affected zone.

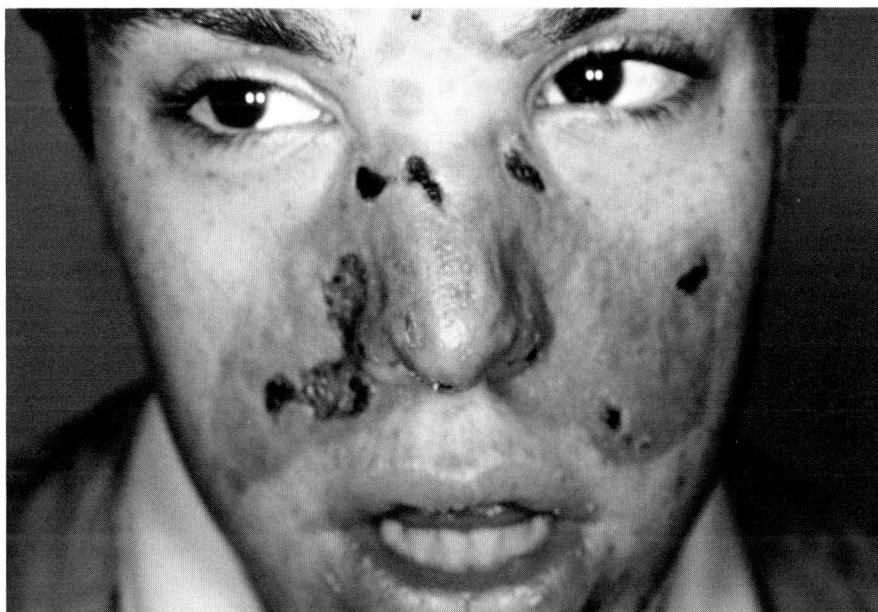

Figure 161. Four weeks after carbon dioxide laser vaporization, the wound has not yet completely healed and there is residual erythema.

Figure 162. Three months following carbon dioxide laser vaporization, there is a return of normal color; although slight textural change is present.

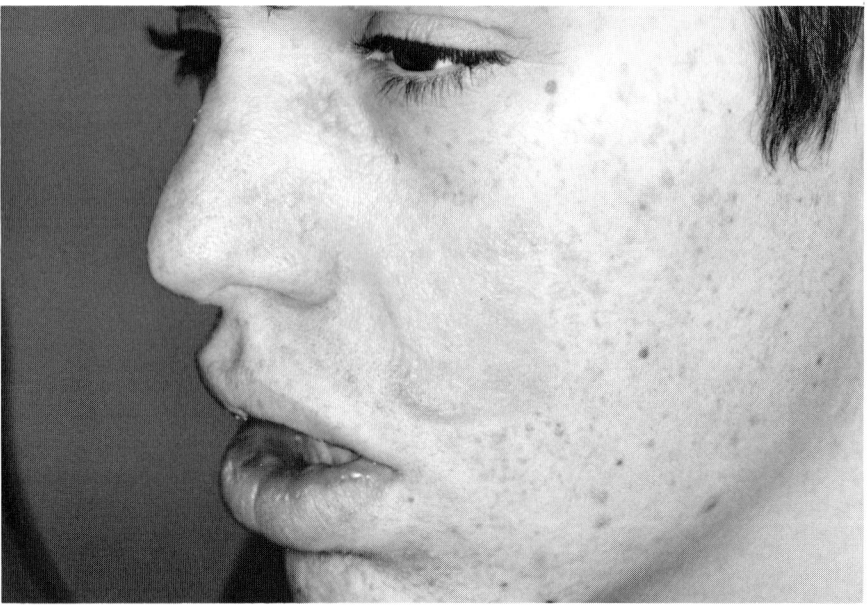

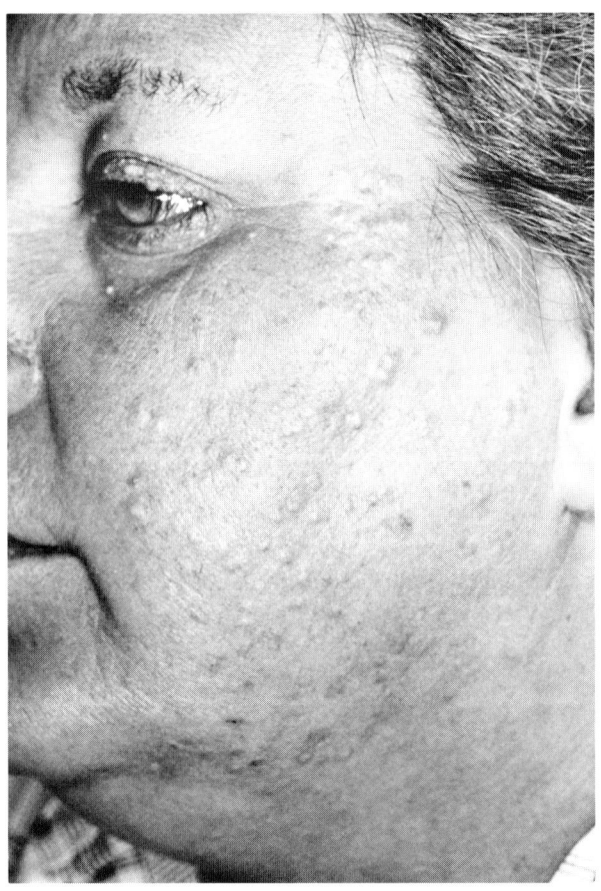

Figure 163. Multiple, small, cystic lesions of vellus hair cysts on the left lateral cheek and temple are identified preoperatively. (See Figures 164–168.)

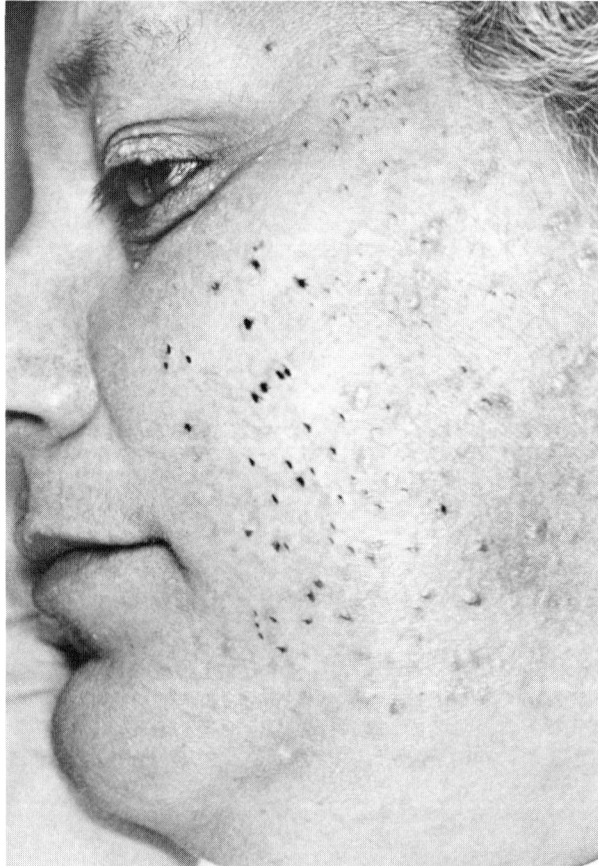

Figure 164. Each lesion is individually marked with a surgical marker.

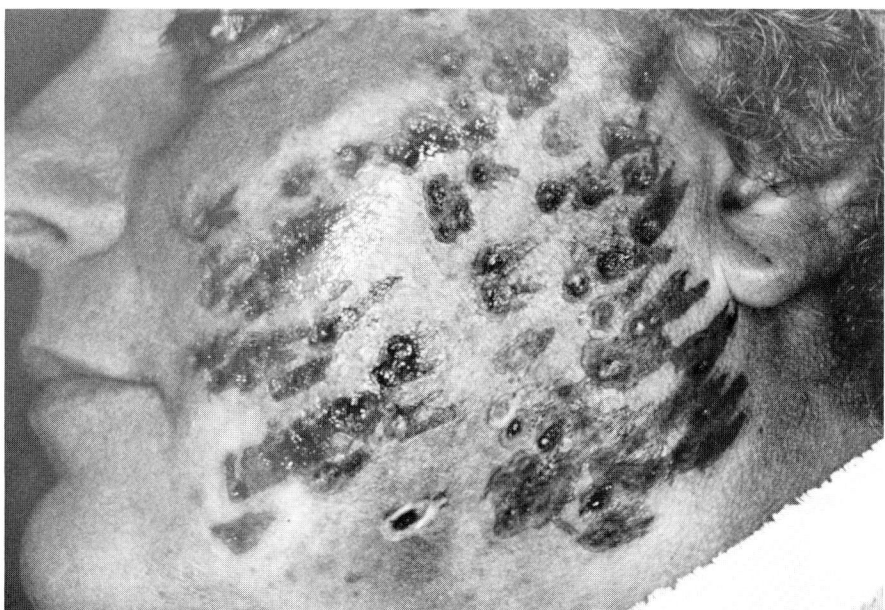

Figure 165. Following vaporization with the carbon dioxide laser, there is minimal bleeding and all cystic structures have been removed.

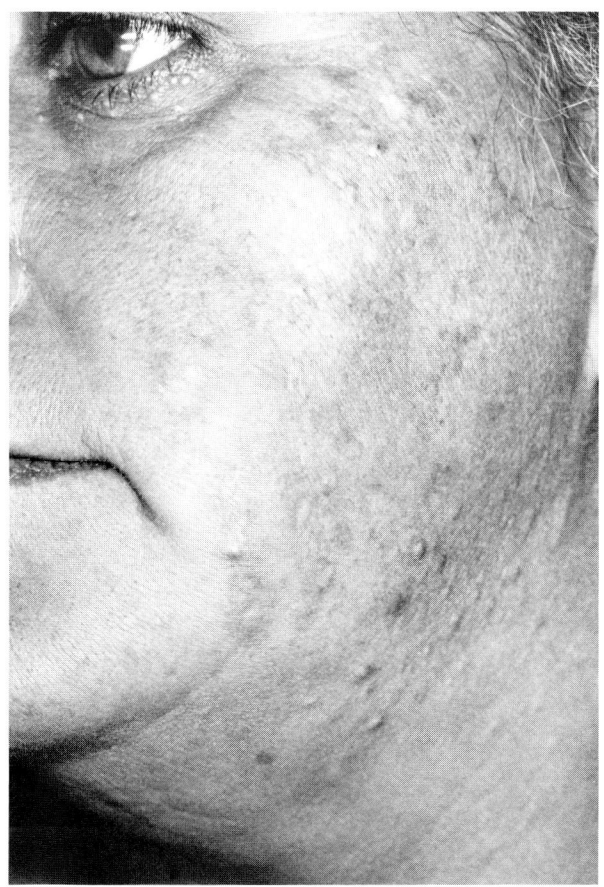

Figure 166. Healing occurs rapidly and by three weeks, the wounds have completely reepithelialized, although residual erythema is seen.

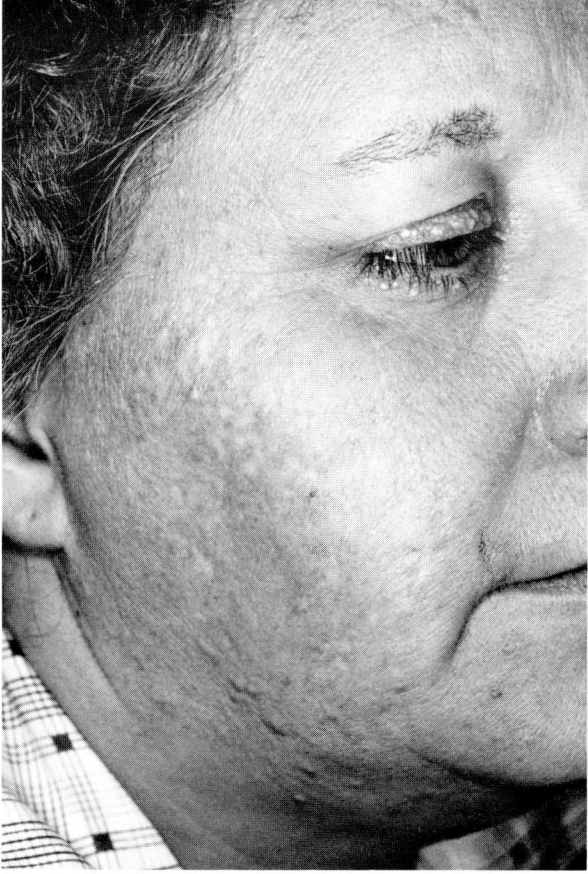

Figure 167. Four months postoperatively there is good texture and nearly normal skin color at the laser treatment sites.

treated in a similar fashion using the defocused carbon dioxide laser vaporization mode of operation. After first marking each lesion (Figure 164) and using local anesthesia, each cystic lesion, usually 1 to 3 mm in diameter and yellow-white in color, is vaporized until the entire cyst wall is removed. By careful observation following cleansing with hydrogen peroxide, the remnants of the cystic structures can usually be seen without difficulty since the carbon dioxide laser permits removal with minimal bleeding (Figure 165). The cysts are then dressed in standard fashion and wound healing occurs over a period of 2 to 3 weeks (Figure 166). Since the depth of involvement in the skin is greater than with any of the clinical lesions described above, there may be some temporary color change, usually in the form of hyperpigmentation which resolves spontaneously in 4 to 6 months in most cases (Figure 167). Because of the large number of lesions in this condition requiring treatment, as well as the potential problem of adverse scarring, it is best to first treat a small test site on a representative area on the face, if possible, prior to initiating treatment of the entire zone of involvement.

MISCELLANEOUS LESIONS TREATED WITH THE CARBON DIOXIDE LASER VAPORIZATION

There are a number of miscellaneous lesions that lend themselves quite readily to treatment with the carbon dioxide laser in its vaporizational mode of operation. A few of the types of lesions that can be satisfactorily treated with the laser include common facial warts, pyogenic granulomas, xanthelasma, acne scars, and granuloma faciale. Each of these clinical conditions will be discussed separately.

Warts

While warts typically occur on the hands and feet, probably as a result of frequency of contact with other infected individuals, they can occur on the face as well. In this situation, they typically appear as flat warts and may be very difficult to treat especially in men who shave every day and inoculate viral particles into noninfected skin (Figures 168–170). While the laser is not considered to be a first mode of treatment for facial

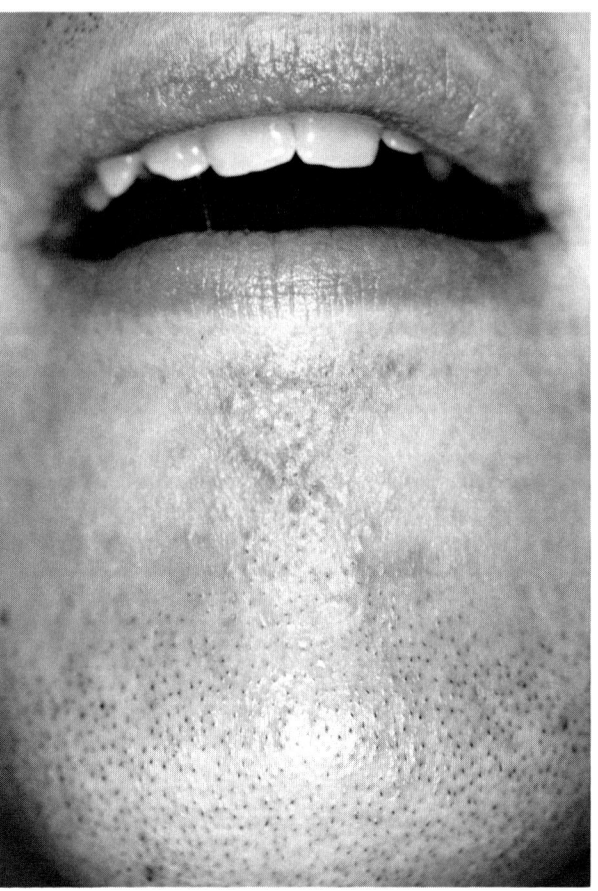

Figure 168. A small number of resistant warts are present on the chin near the lip preoperatively.

warts, it can be used in more refractory cases to provide a successful form of therapy. For this condition, the initial areas of involvement are marked with a surgical marker, local anesthesia is obtained, and each wart is vaporized along with a small zone (1–2 mm) of normal surrounding skin to lessen the likelihood of regrowth from contaminated, but clinically normal appearing surrounding skin. For larger warts of the face, there may be some bubbling of wart tissue as it is vaporized by the carbon dioxide laser beam. This bubbling can offer a rough guideline as to the breadth and depth of this viral infection. If the laser pulses are sufficiently short, 0.05 to 0.1 second pulses, this type of tissue response can be seen. The typical power settings in this situation vary from 4 to 5 watts and a 2 mm defocused beam is utilized to deliver the carbon dioxide energy to the infected epithelium.

After a single layer has been vaporized in this fashion, the infected tissue is cleansed with hydrogen peroxide. Frequently, with light scrub-

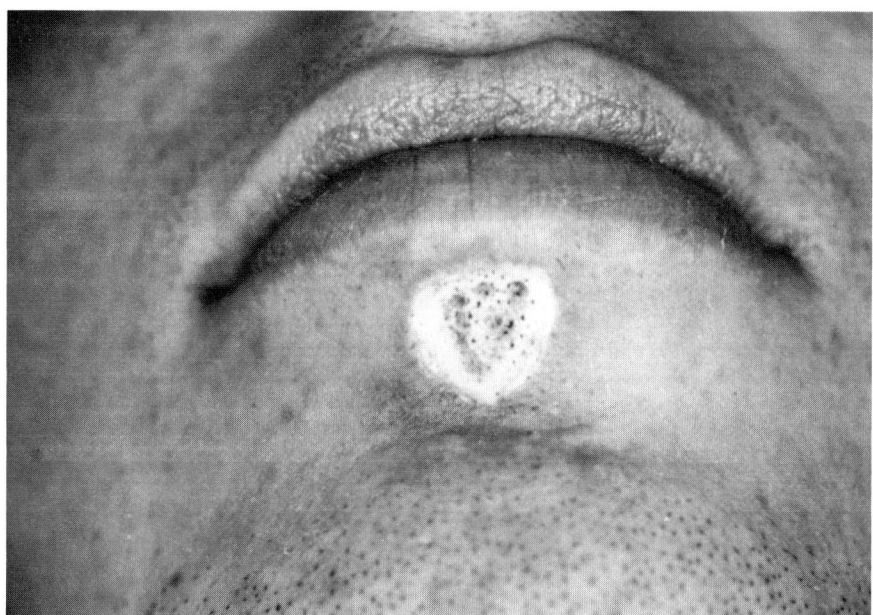

Figure 169. A superficial zone of vaporization has resulted in apparent complete removal of all warts for patient seen in Figure 168.

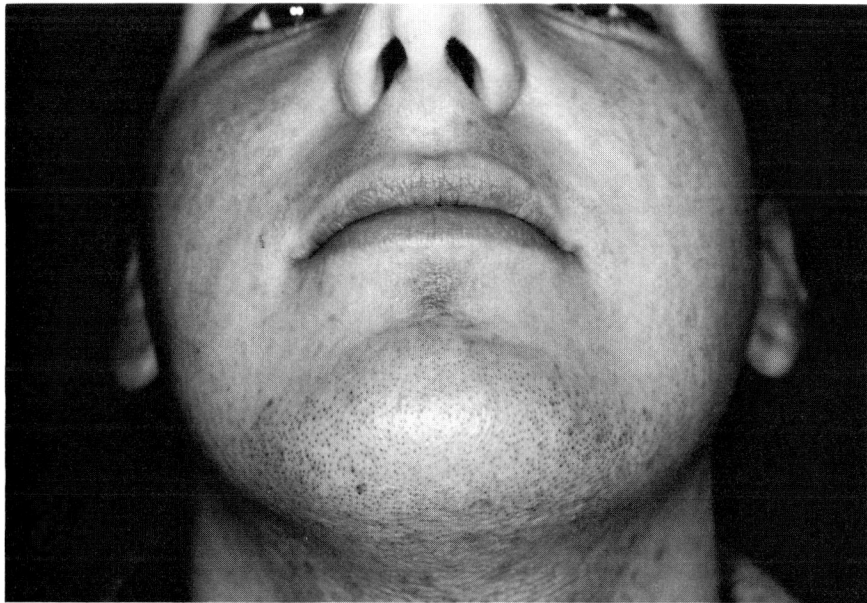

Figure 170. Patient seen in Figure 168 at four weeks postoperatively. There is a slight discoloration noted but no recurrent warts are seen.

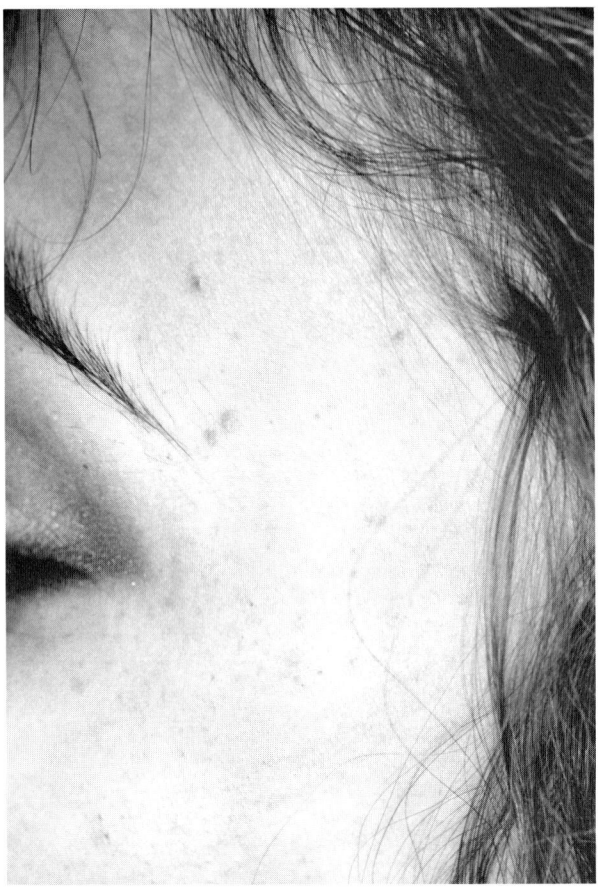

Figure 171. Several small, flat warts are present adjacent to the eyebrow.

minor injury, is not typically seen on the face, but can occur on any part of the body at any site of injury. These lesions typically appear as a bright red or slightly translucent papule of 2 to 8 mm in diameter, surrounded by a thin collar of normal epithelium. These lesions have a high risk of recurrence when treated with standard techniques such as electrocauterization and curettage. Using the carbon dioxide in its vaporization mode, the thermal energy that is created by this laser source is frequently sufficient to heat-seal the proliferating vascular channels and minimize the chances of recurrence. While a guaranteed cure for this condition cannot be promised in all cases treated with the laser, success is very common. Again, because of the depth of involvement of this type of lesion, both scarring and recurrence can be seen after carbon dioxide laser vaporiztion and the patient must be informed of this in advance.

bing, the infected epithelium will separate from the underlying normal tissue at the aparent plane of infection (Figures 171–173). This is the second mechanism by which the laser surgeon can help roughly determine the extent of involvement and improve the success of this procedure. If additional warty tissue is present after cleansing with hydrogen peroxide following initial vaporization, the persistent areas of involvement are retreated in a similar fashion and continued until normal tissue is seen. In most cases, wounds of this type on the face will heal within 7 to 10 days without difficulty. Again, postinflammatory hyperpigmentation and scarring may occur with this technique, but is relatively uncommon. Recurrent growth of facial warts is always possible with any technique, including the laser.

Pyogenic Granuloma

This condition, which represents the formation of hypergranulation tissue usually following

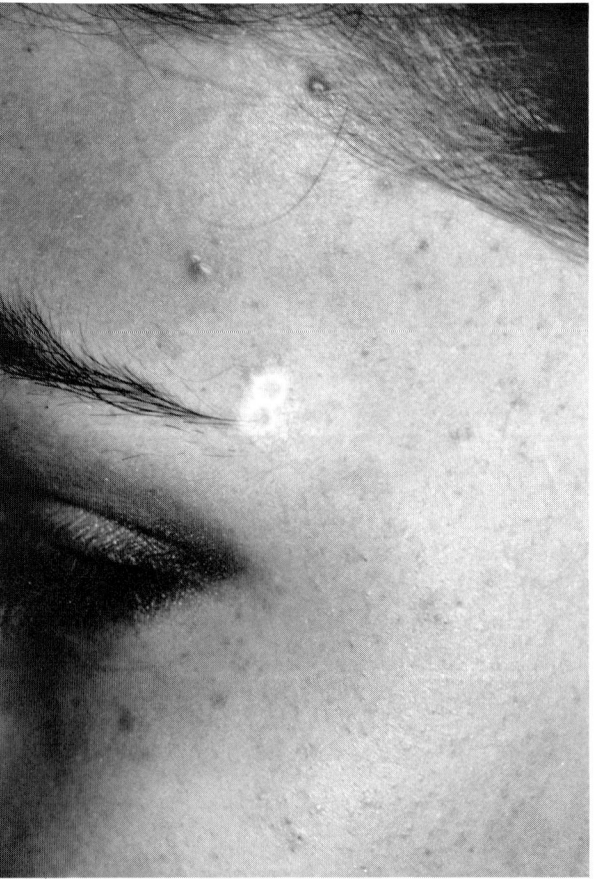

Figure 172. Superficial vaporization has resulted in a complete removal of the warts for patient seen in Figure 171.

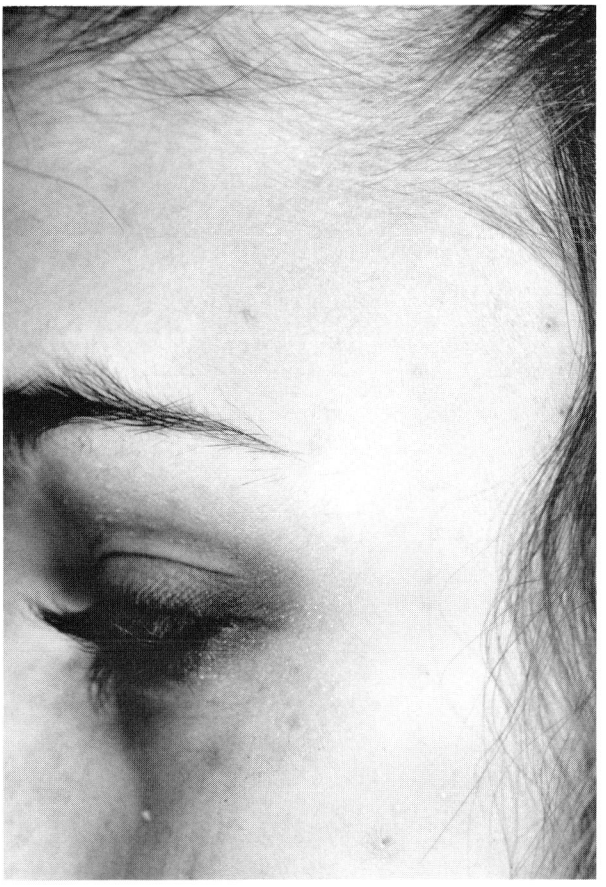

Figure 173. Final cosmetic appearance of patient identified in Figure 171 at four weeks postoperatively shows no residual warts and an inconspicuous treatment site.

Xanthelasma

This condition, which represents deposits of fatty tissue in the periorbital area (Figure 174), may be associated with abnormal levels of cholesterol or triglycerides in the circulation, but may also occur as an inherited trait. The standard types of treatment available for this condition include surgical excision or treatment with a variety of caustic chemicals. The carbon dioxide laser can be utilized to vaporize all of the fatty material from the dermis with precision and at the same time yield an excellent cosmetic result.

In this condition, many laser surgeons will utilize a scleral eyeshield to protect the eye against possible inadvertent injury from contact with the laser beam. After obtaining local anesthesia and marking the zone of involvement, the abnormal tissue is vaporized using 4 watts of power, a 2 mm beam diameter, and pulses of laser energy of 0.2 to 0.5 seconds in duration. After the entire zone has been treated in this fashion, the surface char is removed with hydrogen peroxide and the base examined for presence of additional fatty tissue (Figure 175). If additional fatty material can be visualized, usually by its different color or texture compared to the normal surrounding skin, these remaining areas of involvement are treated in a similar fashion until complete removal is ensured. Standard dressings are then applied, and with standard wound care the patient will

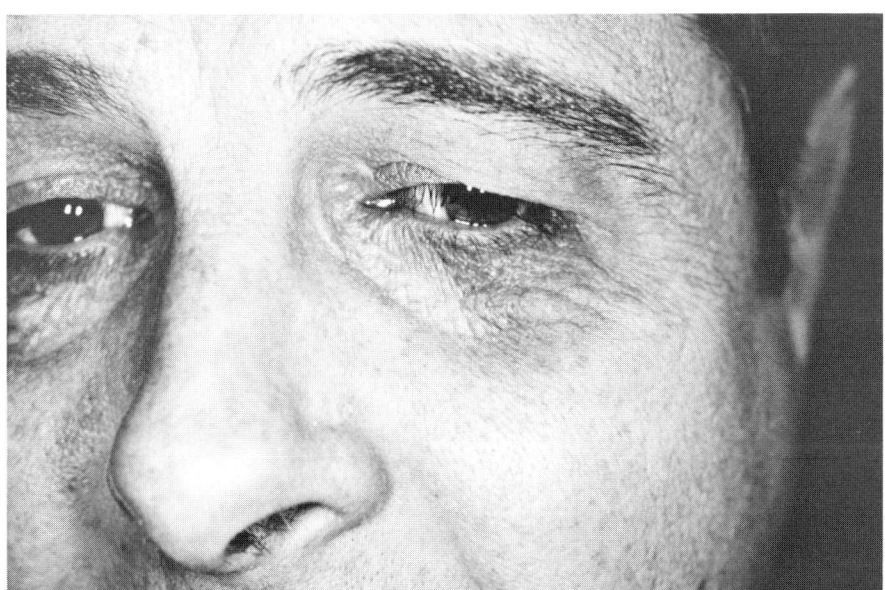

Figure 174. Prominent xanthelasma and periorbital hyperpigmentation are seen preoperatively.

Figure 175. Superficial vaporization of the area of xanthoma has been performed under local anesthesia for patient seen in Figure 174.

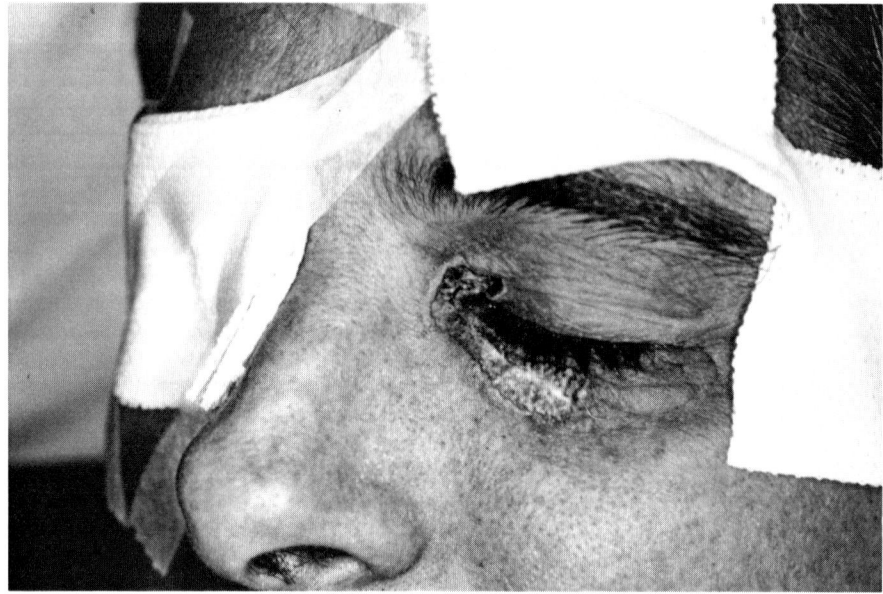

typically heal in 7 to 10 days. One of the pluses of the carbon dioxide laser in this technique is that most patients have minimal postoperative pain, edema, and ecchymosis and the final cosmetic result is excellent (Figure 176). If the deposition of fatty material extends close to the ciliary margin and there is a concern about possible perforation, an additional zone of safety can be attained by the infiltration of sterile normal saline under the treatment site which will act to absorb carbon dioxide laser energy that might otherwise pene-

trate through to deeper vital structures. This simple maneuver can allow precision, complete removal and, yet, total safety in the treatment of this relatively common disorder.

Acne Scars

While this technique is largely experimental in nature, the carbon dioxide laser has been used in the treatment of small pitted facial acne scars

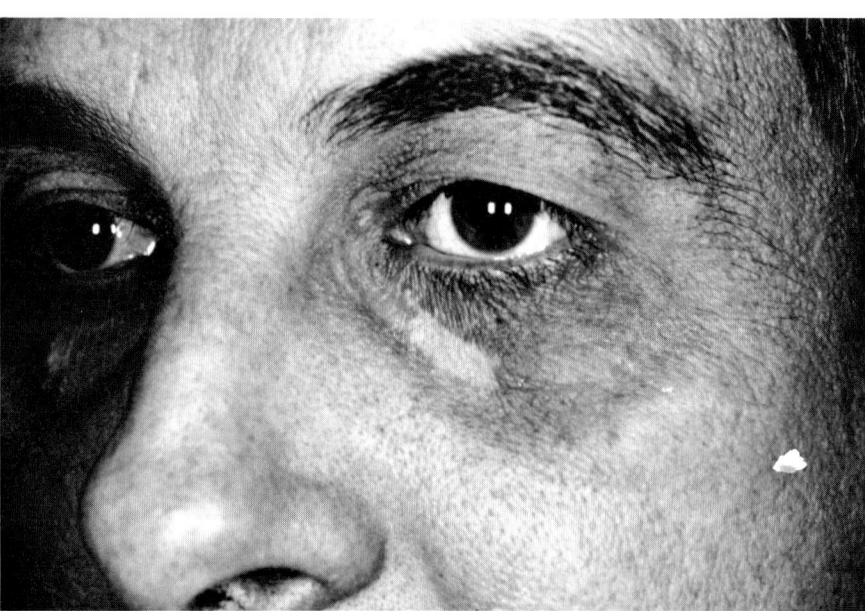

Figure 176. Final appearance of patient identified in Figure 174 six weeks postoperatively showing no recurrence of the xanthelasma and improvement in the hyperpigmentation at the treatment site compared to the normal hyperpigmentation seen.

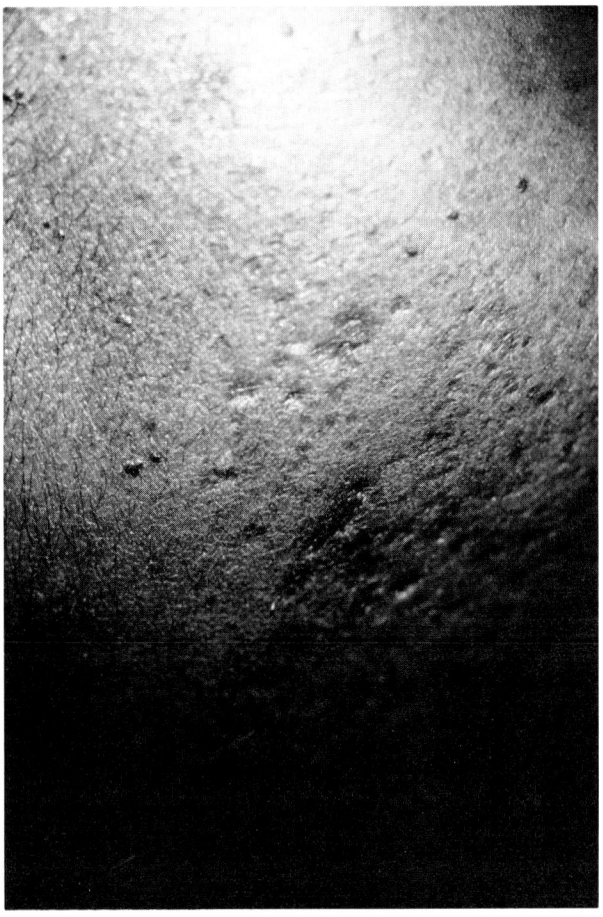

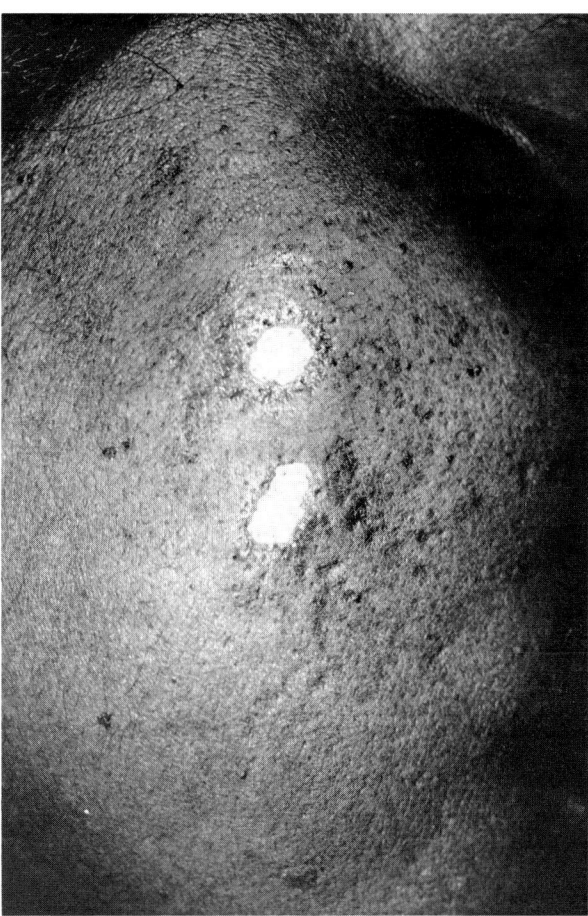

Figure 177. Several small deeply pitted scars from acne are present preoperatively on the right cheek.

Figure 178. Same patient as in Figure 177. After vaporization, the contours of the scar have been softened.

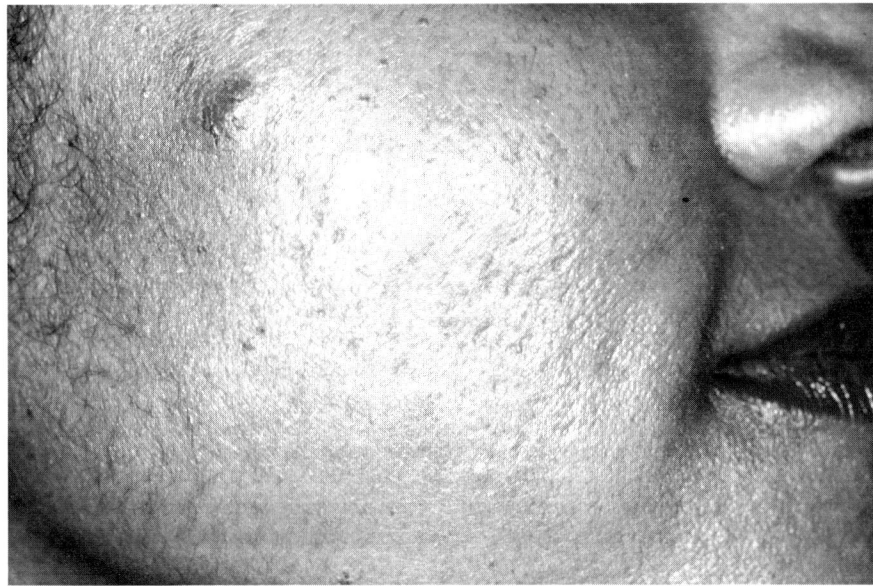

Figure 179. Six weeks after laser abrasion, the acne scars are substantially improved and the cosmetic results are excellent for patient seen in Figure 177.

(Figure 177). This technique is sometimes known as a laserabrasion and, although performed on a much smaller scale, is similar to that technique described above for treating diffuse adenoma sebaceum.

In this procedure, a small test area is first treated to evaluate healing and effectiveness. Once this has been performed and good results achieved, the pitted scars to be treated are marked with a surgical marker and local anesthesia is obtained. With a 1 mm diameter laser beam, 4 watts of power, and pulse duration of 0.1 to 0.2 seconds, the scar is vaporized (Figure 178) so that the sharp contours are eliminated and the defect blends in more readily with the surrounding skin (Figure 179).

Using a computer-directed laser beam and a micromanipulator, full face laserabrasions for acne scarring have now been performed. Since the curved contours of the face can interfere with precise vaporization of large surfaces, additional refinements will be required before this technique is widely used.

Granuloma Faciale

An uncommon, but not rare, inflammatory condition of the skin is known as granuloma faciale. In this condition, localized deposits of inflammatory cells and granulomas develop on ex-

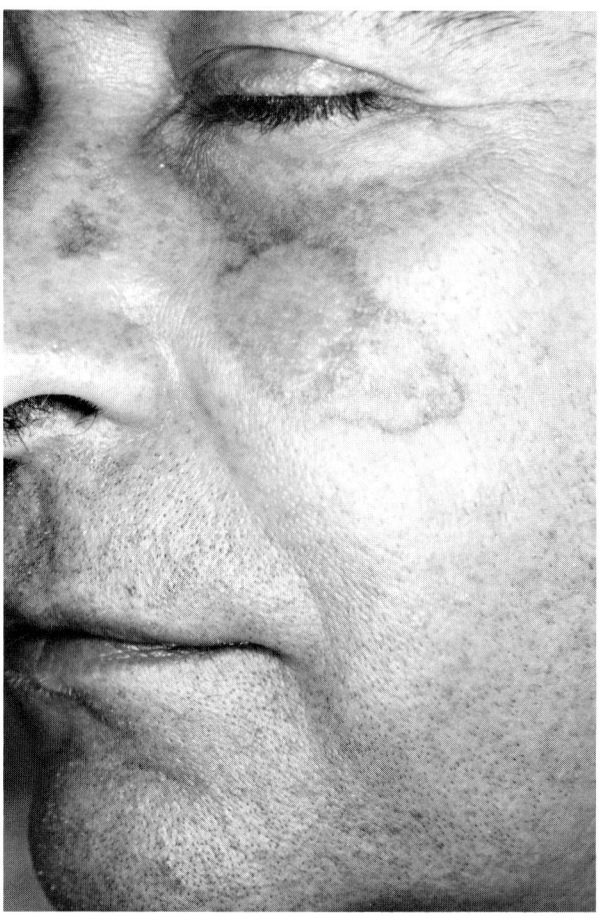

Figure 180. Large zone of induration and hyperpigmentation is present on the left superior cheek preoperatively. (See Figures 181–185.)

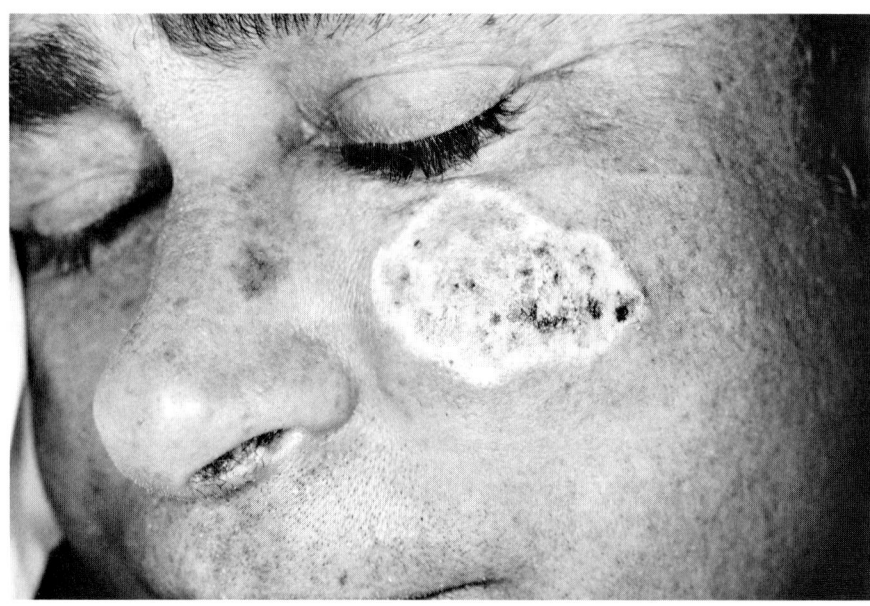

Figure 181. Vaporization with the carbon dioxide laser has removed all granulomatous tissue.

posed portions of the face (Figure 180). These bluish-brown discolored plaques of 1 to 8 cm in size may be the source of significant cosmetic impairment. While surgical excision has been employed, and argon laser phototherapy has also been used, recurrences are common.

The carbon dioxide laser can be used to vaporize these granulomas with tremendous success (Figures 181 and 182). The technique employed in the treatment of this condition is similar to that described above. The affected area (Figure 183) is first outlined with a surgical marker and local anesthesia is obtained by intradermal injection of 1% lidocaine with epinephrine 1 : 200,000. The area to be treated is vaporized with laser settings of 4 to 5 watts, a 2 mm beam, and continuous discharge. After the entire treatment area has been vaporized, the surface char is cleansed with hydrogen peroxide and the base of the wound is then examined for persistence of abnormal tissue (Figure 184). In this case, the granulomatous process appears as irregular micropapules that are slightly lighter in color than the normal surrounding dermis.

If persistent granulomas are seen after the first treatment pass, a second layer is vaporized in similar fashion. This is continued until all abnormal tissue has been removed. The wound is allowed to heal by second intention and good cosmetic results can be obtained usually within 2 to 3 weeks (Figure 185). While recurrences may, indeed, happen, it seems to be less likely than

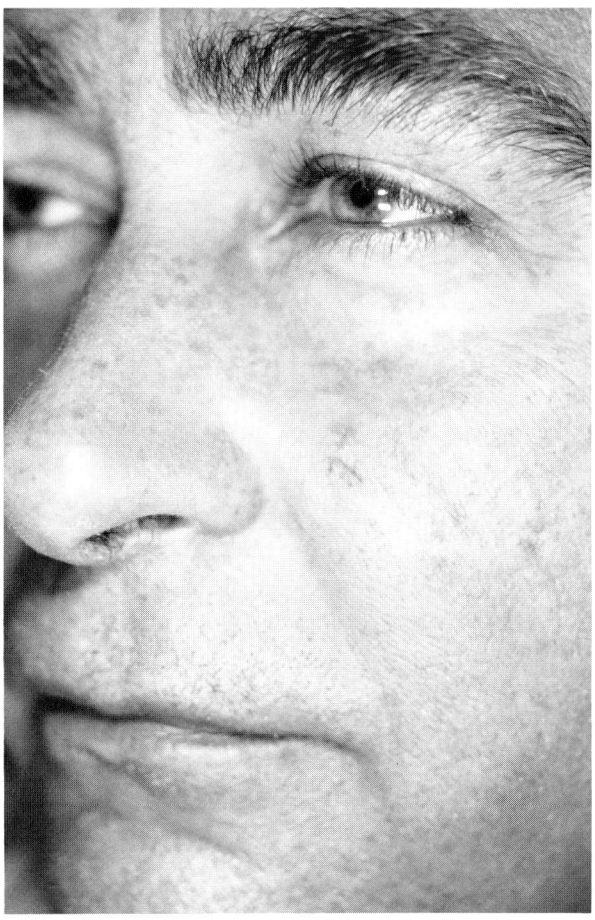

Figure 182. Cosmetic appearance obtained at three weeks shows rapid healing, no evidence of persistent granulomas, and a cosmetically acceptable scar.

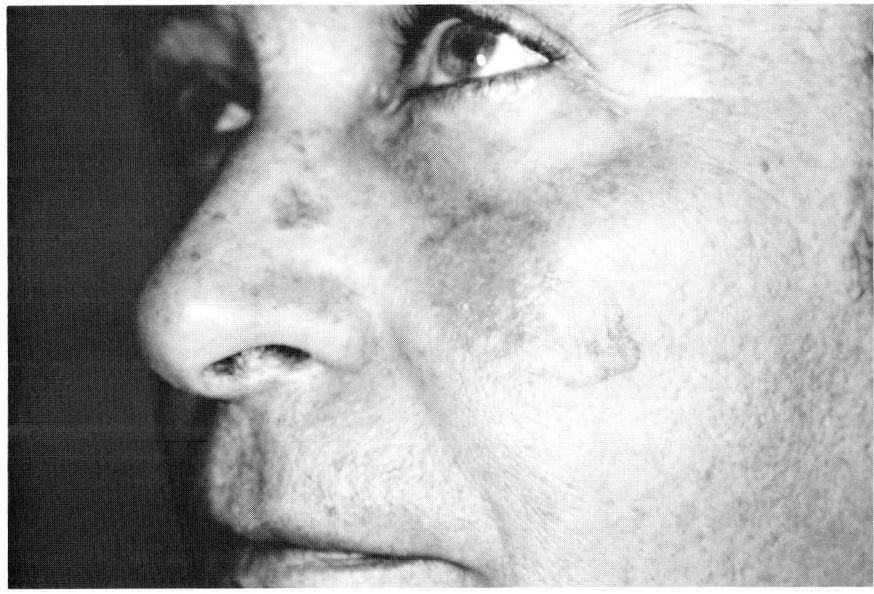

Figure 183. A similar zone of granuloma faciale is present on the nasal bridge.

Figure 184. Superficial vaporization of this zone has removed all granulomas.

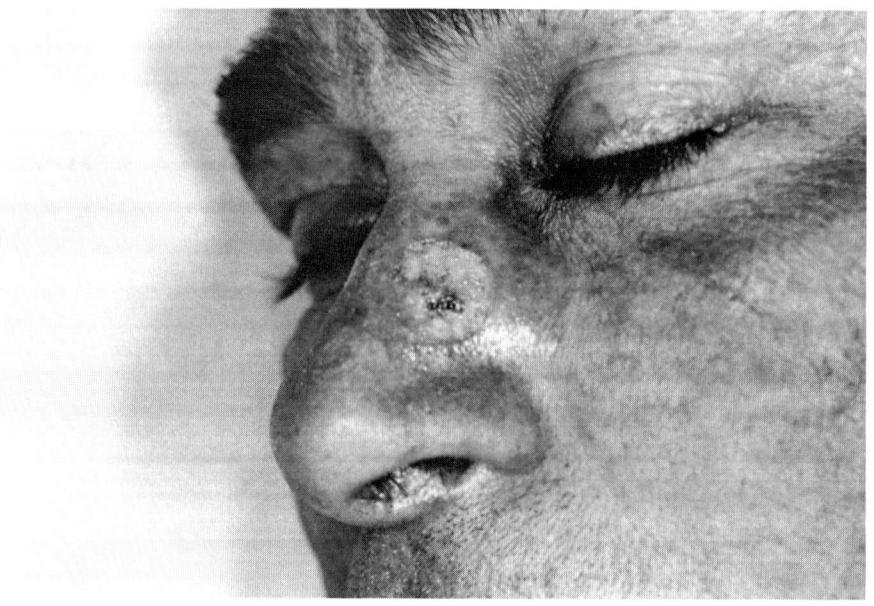

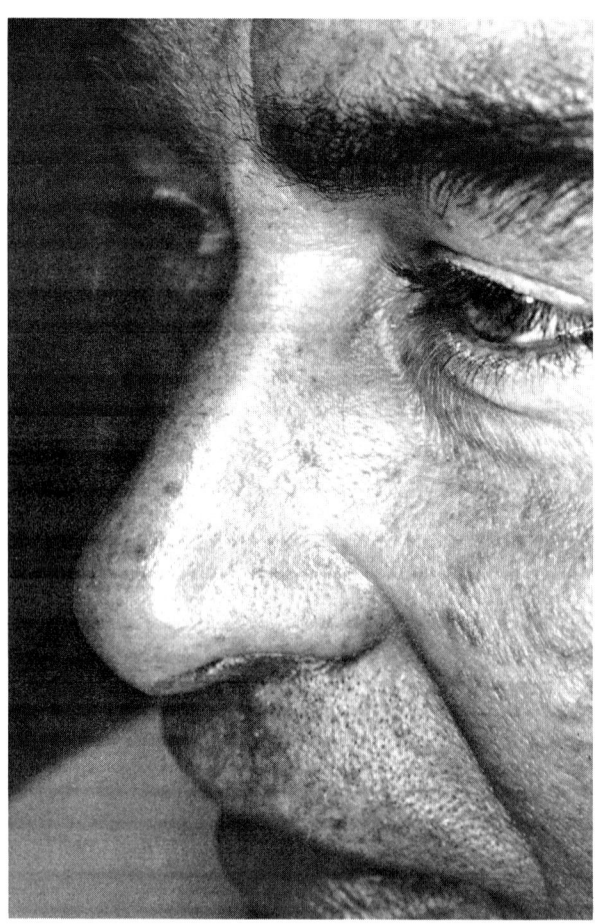

Figure 185. Complete healing has occurred by three weeks with residual erythema but excellent texture and contours are seen.

with the more traditional techniques. This may be due to the slight thermal heating of tissue around the zone of vaporization that causes subclinical destruction of the inflammatory cells.

OTHER VASCULAR CONDITIONS TREATED WITH LASER VAPORIZATION

While the argon laser has certainly proven to be the most useful laser for the treatment of vascular conditions, the carbon dioxide laser, as previously discussed in the treatment of angiomas, can also be used to treat some vascular conditions successfully. Two of these conditions include solar telangiectasia (Figures 186 – 189) and arteriovenous fistula (Figures 190 – 192). Each of these conditions may occur on the exposed portions of the face and neck. The treatment for each of these conditons is similar to that described above. The areas of abnormal tissue are vaporized under local anesthesia with similar laser parameters. The thermal interaction of the carbon dioxide laser energy with the surrounding tissue is probably responsible for the improvement seen in each of these two conditions. While recurrences may develop from subsequent sunlight exposure or trauma, the cosmetic result following laser ablation with the vaporizational technique is usually satisfactory.

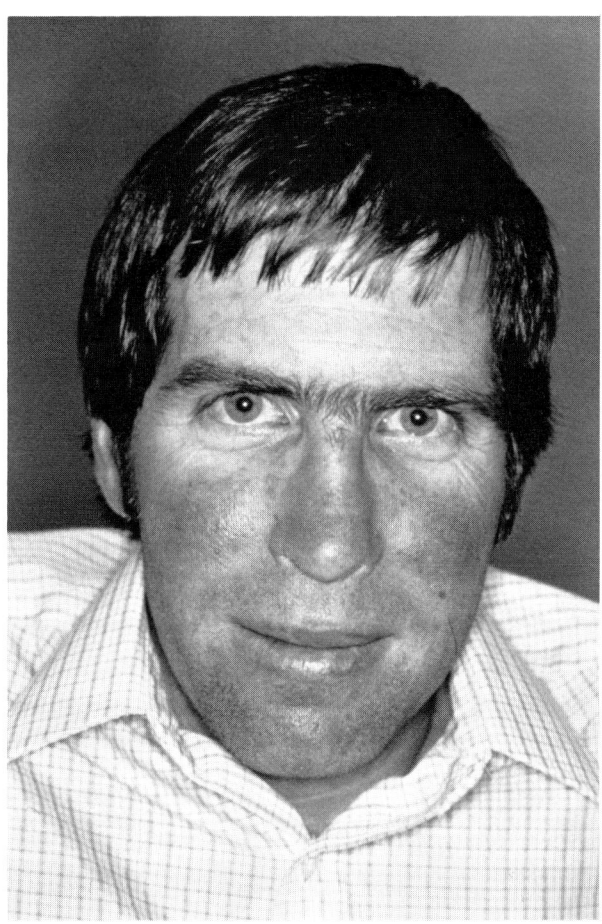

Figure 186. Severe solar telangiectasias of both cheeks is seen preoperatively. (See Figures 187–189.)

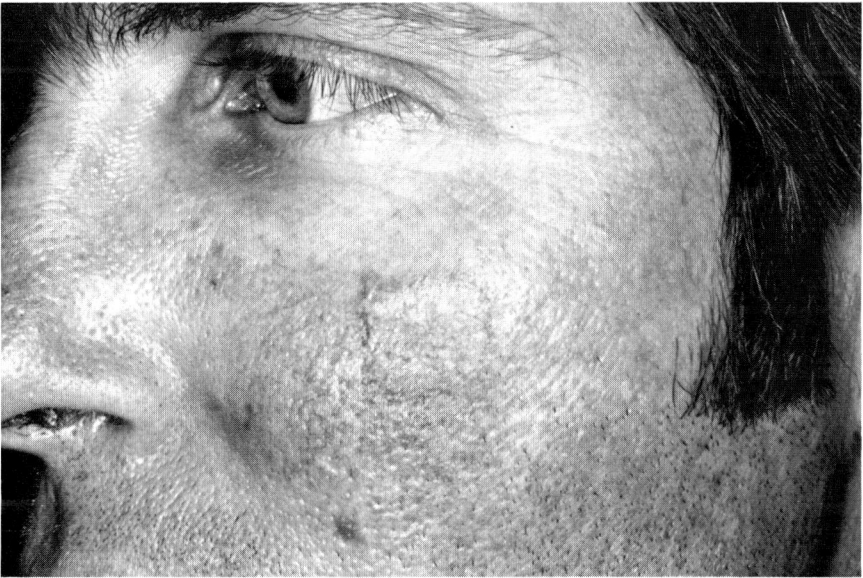

Figure 187. A small, square, carbon dioxide laser test site is outlined with a surgical marker.

Figure 188. The clinical appearance immediately after carbon dioxide laser vaporization has been performed.

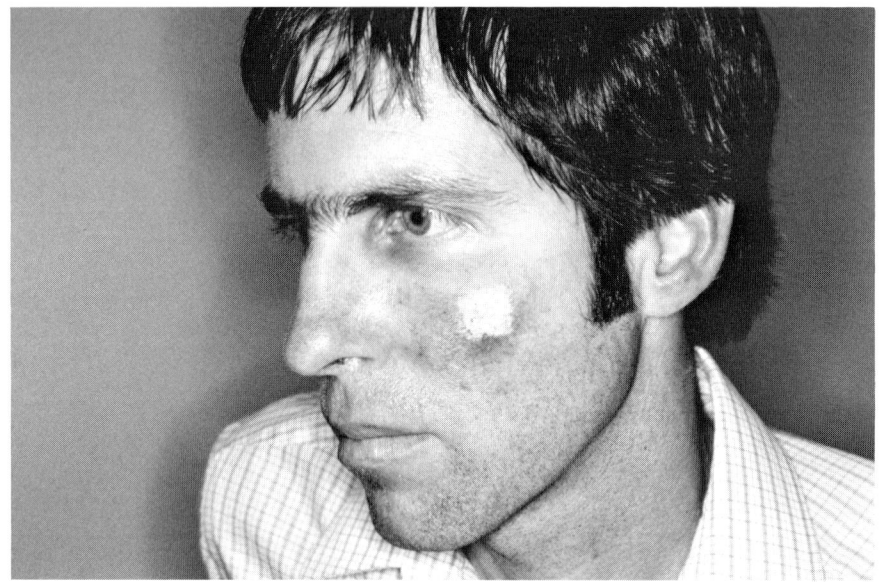

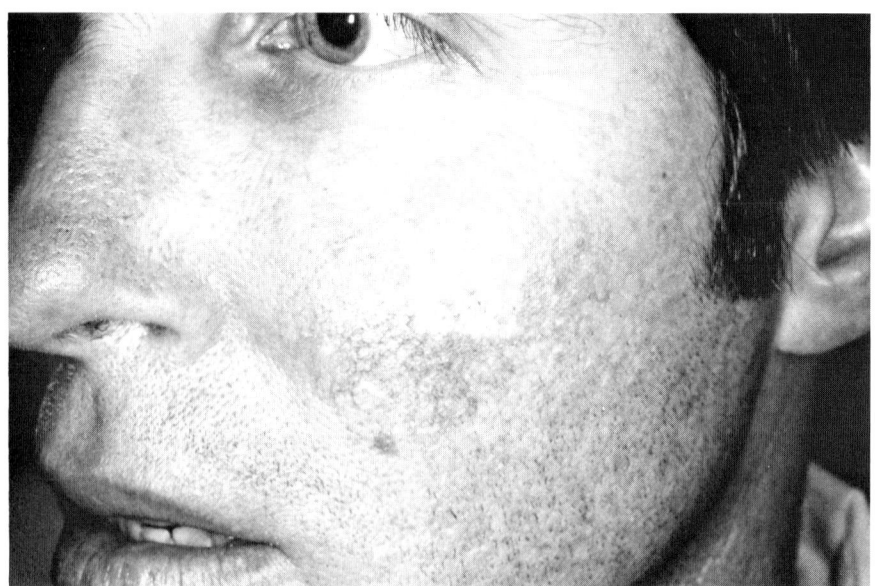

Figure 189. Cosmetic results obtained four months post-laser treatment showing no recurrent growth of the telangiectasias and excellent cosmetic result.

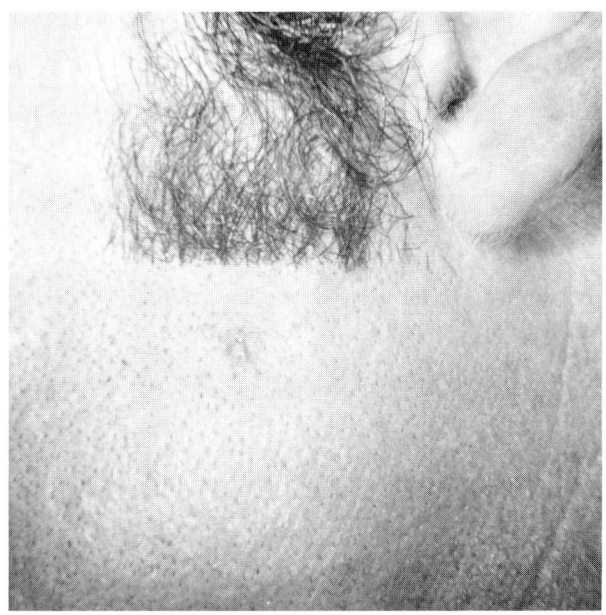

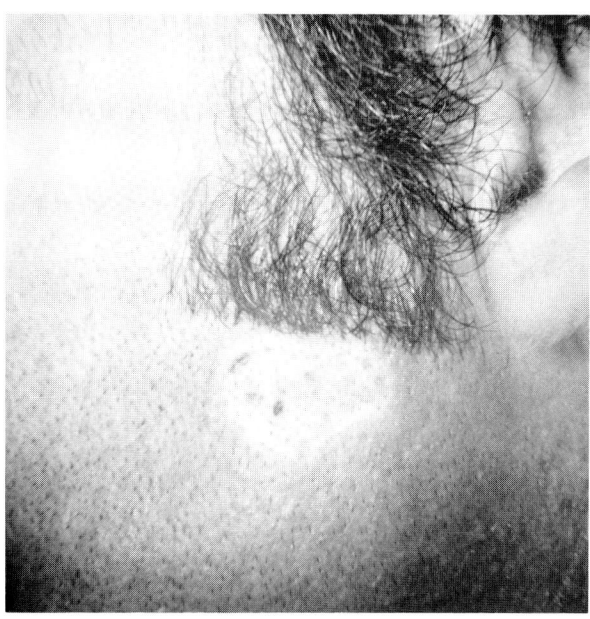

Figure 190. A small, traumatic arteriovenous fistula is seen on the left lateral cheek preoperatively. (See Figures 191 and 192.)

Figure 191. The extent of this vascular collection can be seen after carbon dioxide laser vaporization of the affected zone has been performed.

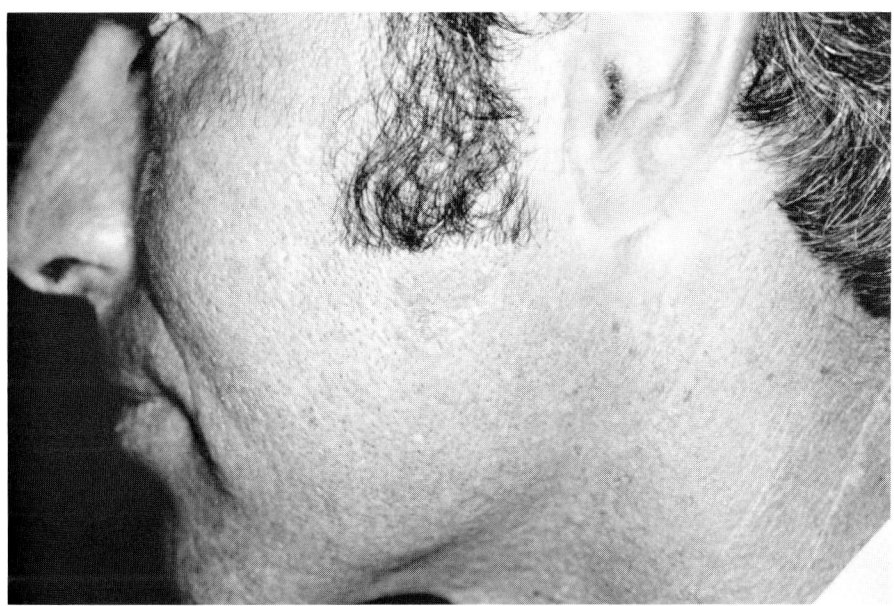

Figure 192. Slight erythema and some textural change is present four weeks postoperatively but no recurrent vascular growth is identified.

LASER VAPORIZATION OF RHINOPHYMA

The diffuse enlargement of the soft tissues of the nose, typically seen in men beyond the age of 40, is known as rhinophyma (Figure 193). While there are many different surgical techniques utilized in the treatment of this disfiguring condition, the carbon dioxide laser does offer some additional advantages. It can be used to vaporize the affected zones of involvement or can be used initially as a light scalpel to roughly sculpt the contours of the soft tissue to the approximate shape and then use the vaporization mode to precisely remove thinner layers of tissue from the hypertrophic mass.

In this procedure, distortion of the nose caused by local anesthesia is avoided by performing nerve blocks. This is done with 1% lidocaine with epinephrine 1 : 100,000. If possible, the patient should provide a photograph taken before the soft tissue enlargement occurred to permit the surgeon to more closely reapproximate the normal size and shape of the nose. Once the determination has been made as to the volume of tissue that needs to be removed, either vaporization alone or excision with the laser followed by vaporization is employed.

Most typically, if only a small volume of tissue is to be removed, the laser is set for vaporization at 4 to 6 watts of power and a 2 mm beam is used with a continuous discharge mode. The entire treatment site is vaporized (Figure 194) at these parameters and the base is carefully cleansed with hydrogen peroxide (Figures 195 – 197). The wound is examined to estimate how much additional soft tissue must be removed. There is usually no bleeding with this procedure as compared with the traditional techniques in which dermabrasion causes the spattering of blood over the entire operative field as well as the surgeon and assistants. Since there is no bleeding, the sur-

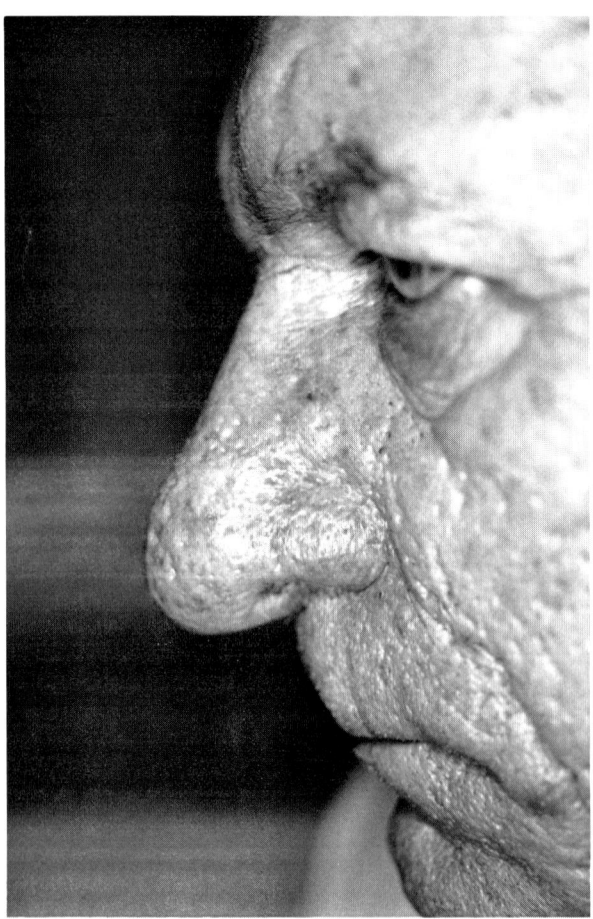

Figure 193. Irregular soft tissue enlargement of the nose is present.

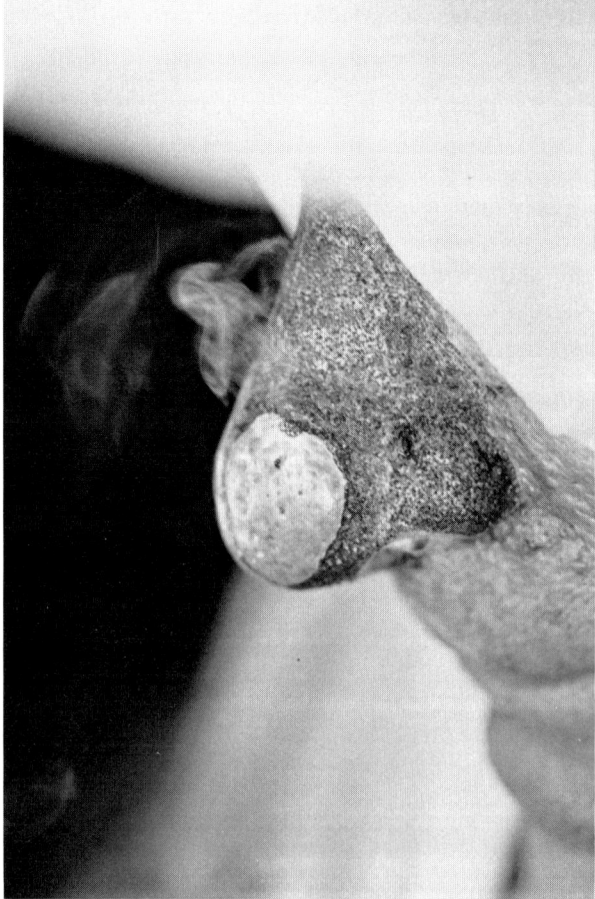

Figure 194. Vaporization has begun at the nasofacial sulcus and is continuing toward the nasal tip.

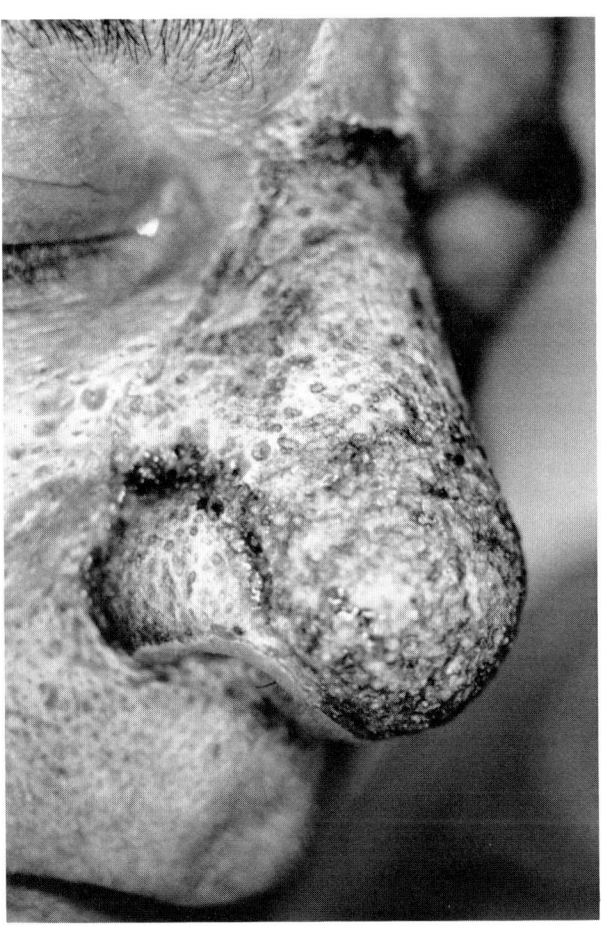

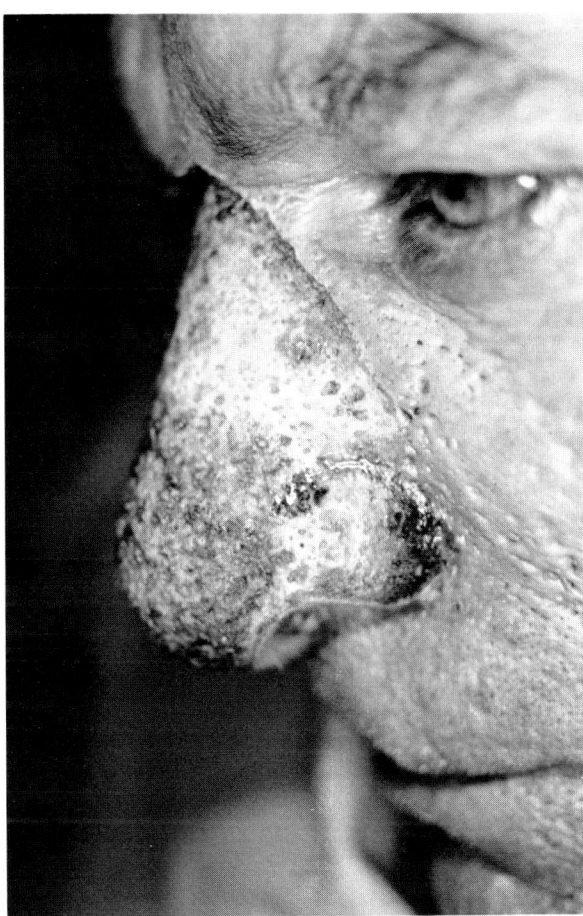

Figure 195. After vaporization of the entire zone has been completed, cleansing with hydrogen peroxide removes all surface char from the right side of the nose. (See Figures 196 and 197.)

Figure 196. Following carbon dioxide laser vaporization, the char has been removed from the left side of the nose.

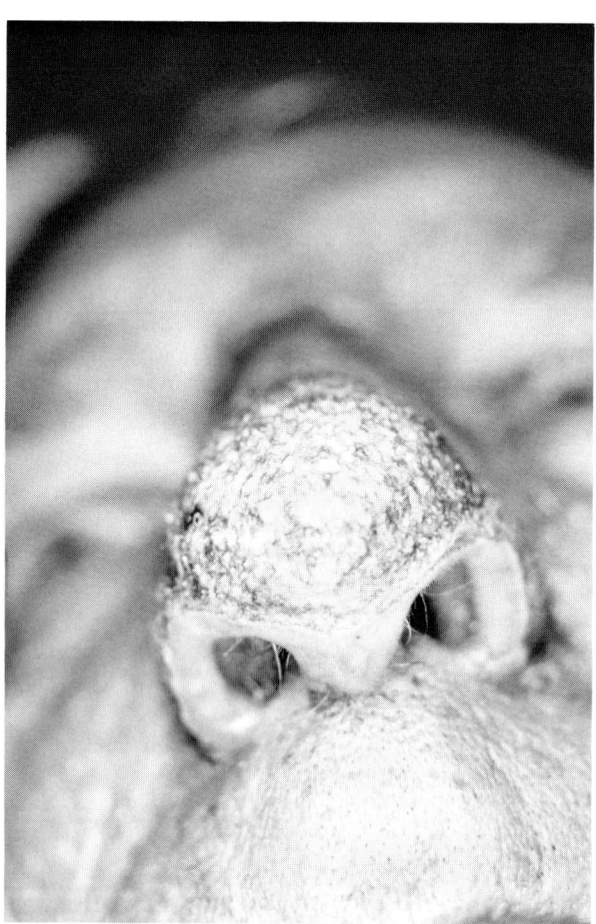

Figure 197. Following carbon dioxide laser vaporization, the char has been removed from the nasal tip.

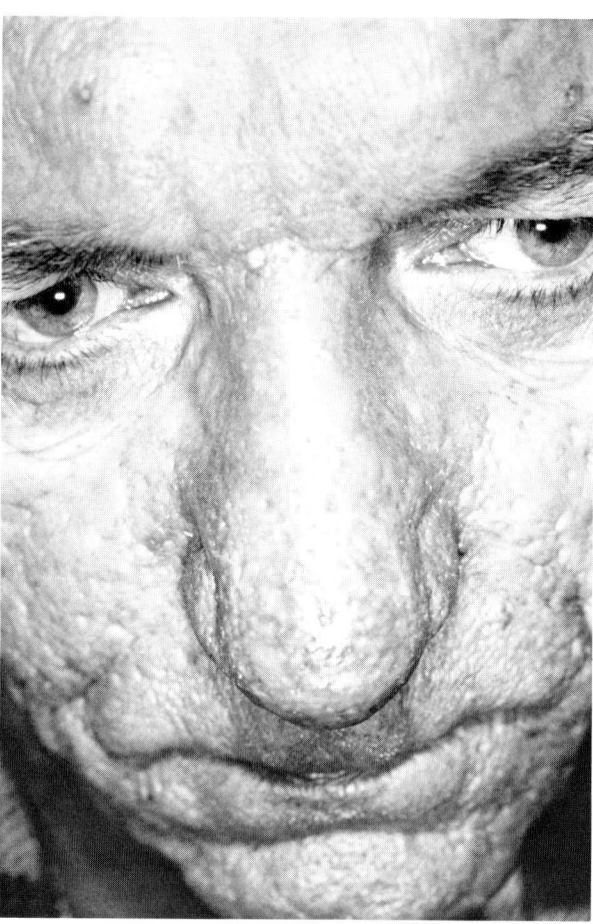

Figure 198. Frontal view of patient shown on Figure 193 six weeks postoperatively showing complete healing, reduction in the size of the nose and an improved texture.

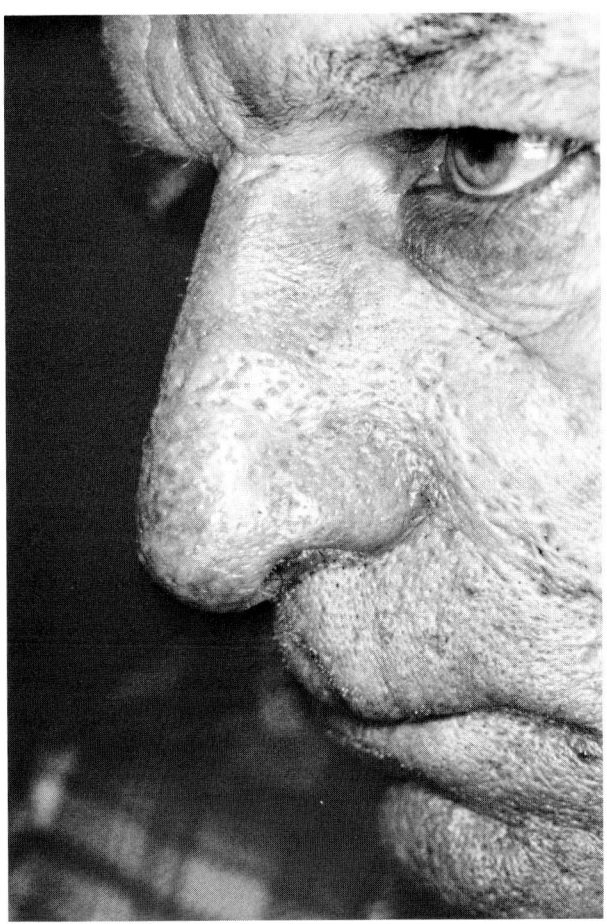

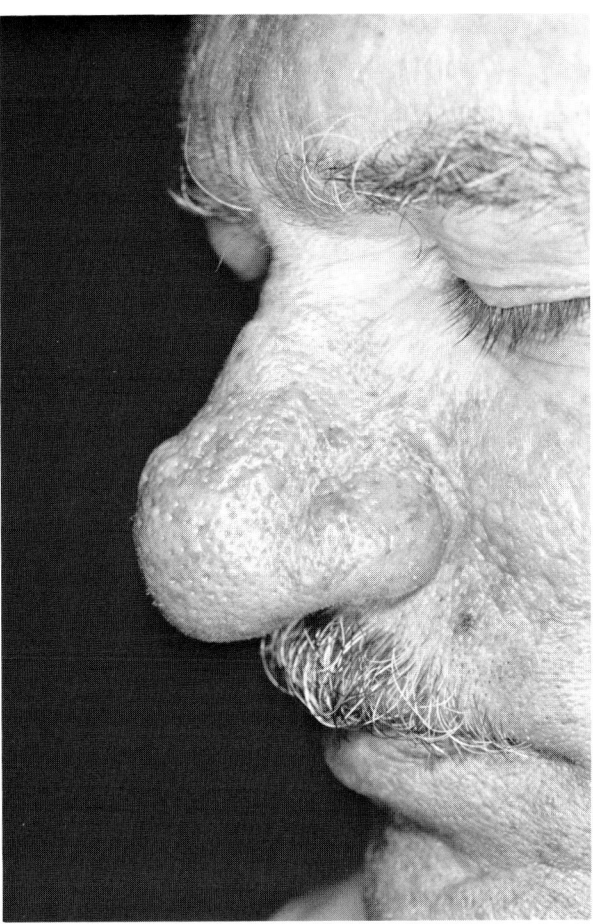

Figure 199. Lateral view of the same patient shown in Figure 198 six weeks postoperatively showing the reduction in size and improved texture.

Figure 201. Preoperative appearance of patient with significant rhinophyma. (See Figures 202–206.)

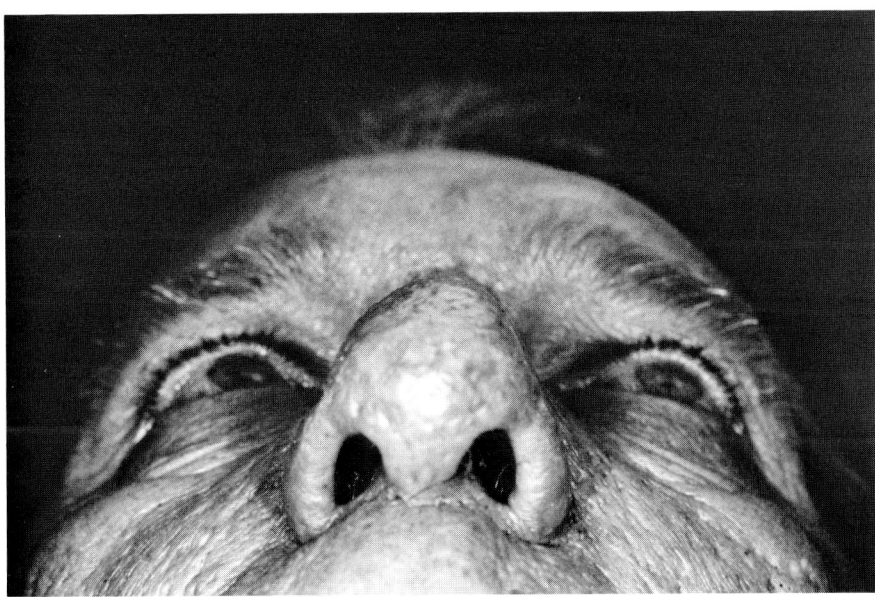

Figure 200. Inferior view of patient demonstrated in Figures 198 and 199 showing reduction in size of the nasal tip and excellent texture.

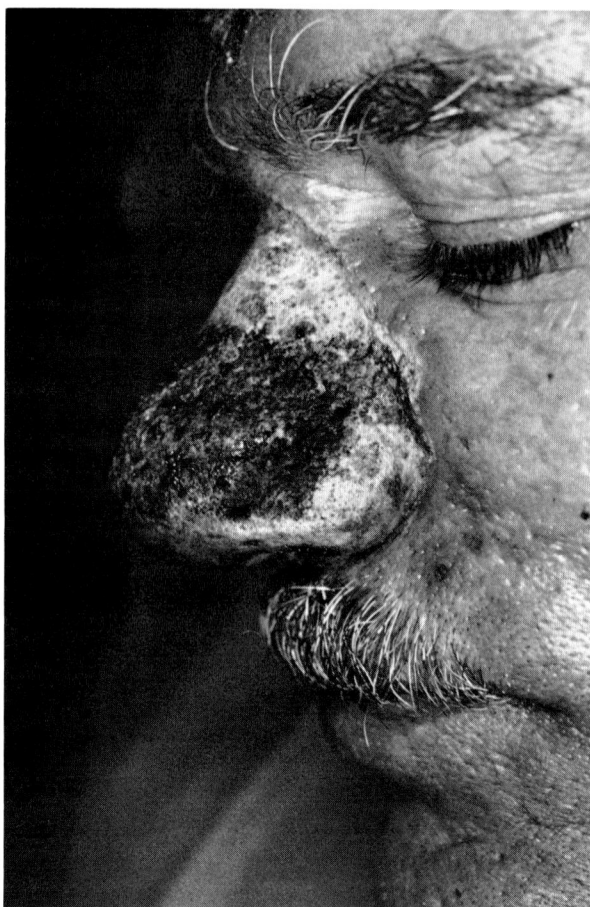

Figure 202. Clinical appearance immediately after carbon dioxide laser vaporization has been performed.

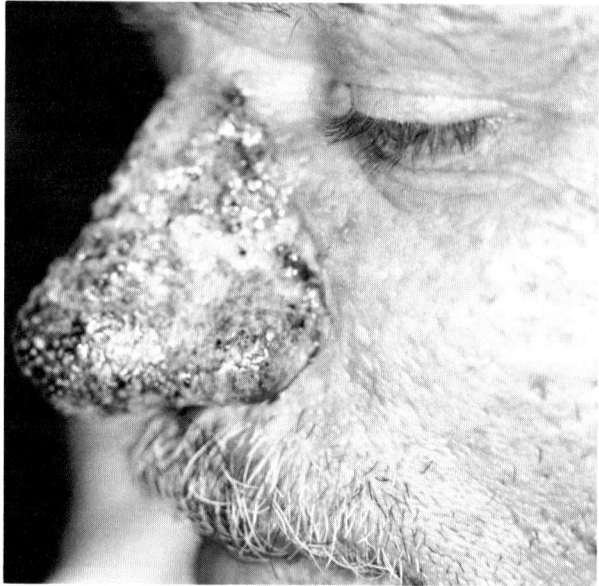

Figure 203. Superficial crusting is present at one week postoperatively.

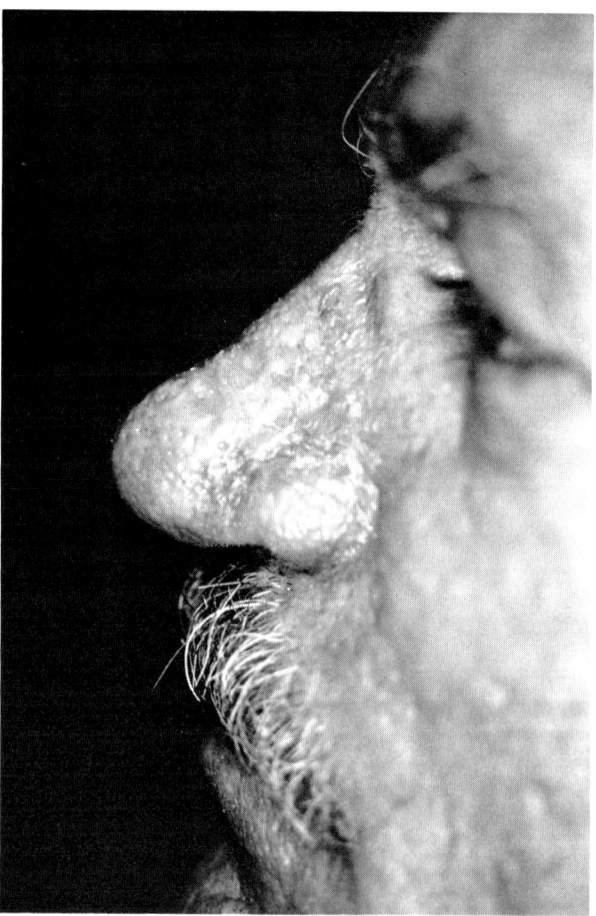

Figure 204. Slight erythema and only small focal areas of the wound require epithelialization by three weeks postoperatively.

geon can more accurately estimate the amount of soft tissue removed as well as the possible need for additional treatment of persistent areas of excess soft tissue.

If focal areas of hypertrophy are present, these can be shaved flush with the surrounding skin using the focused carbon dioxide laser beam. Then using the defocused mode, additional thinner layers of tissue can be precisely removed to produce the normal contours of the nose. Once all excess soft tissue has been removed, a sterile dressing is applied. While there may be some exudate from the surface over the first 72 hours, pain is usually minimal and postoperative bleeding is not a problem. In many cases, patients can frequently return to work within 72 hours even though a dressing may be required. Reepithelialization occurs from the remaining portions of the pilosebaceous structures and is oftentimes complete in 7 to 10 days (Figures 198–200). While

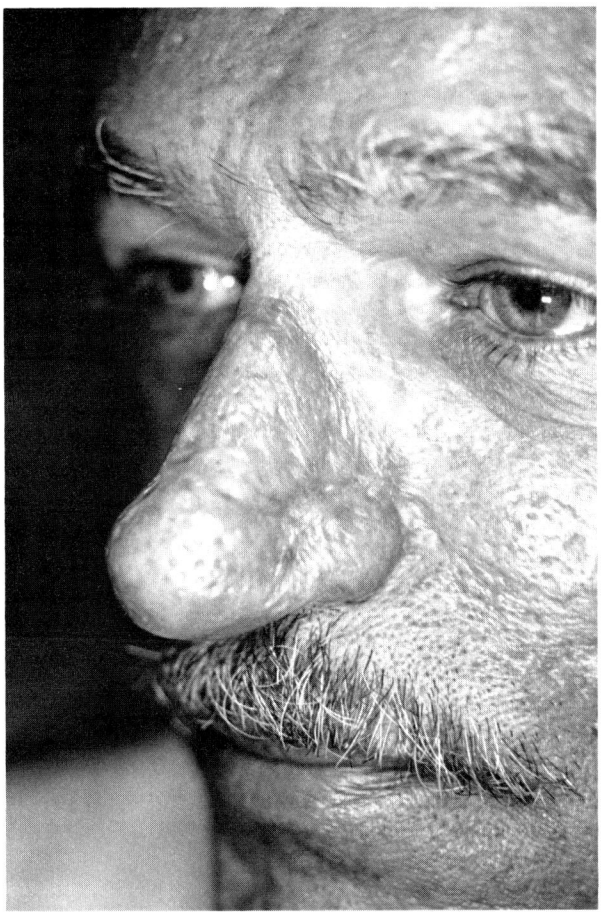

Figure 205. Appearance of the wound showing slight erythema six weeks postoperatively, but an excellent cosmetic result with reduction in size and an improvement in both texture and contour have been obtained.

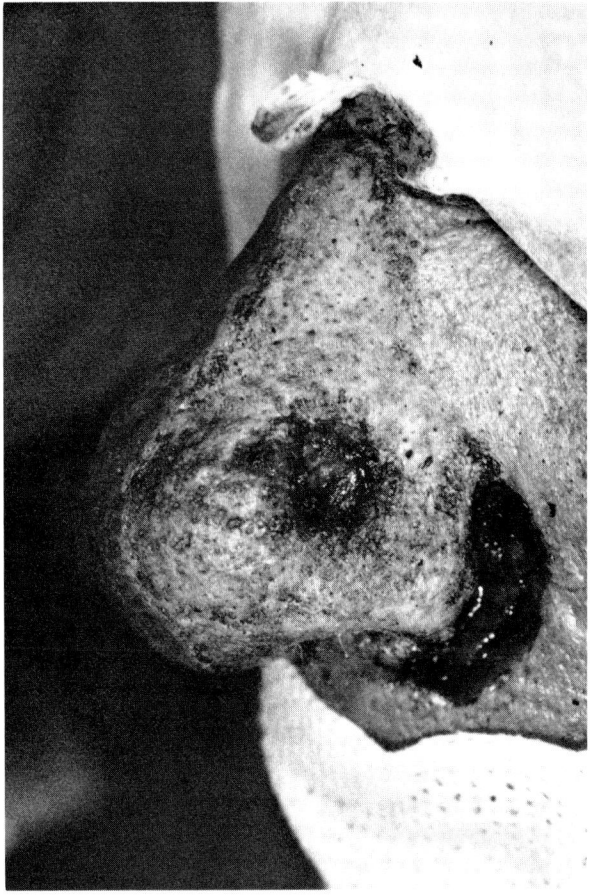

Figure 207. Clinical appearance immediately after laser vaporization of the focal areas of hypertrophy.

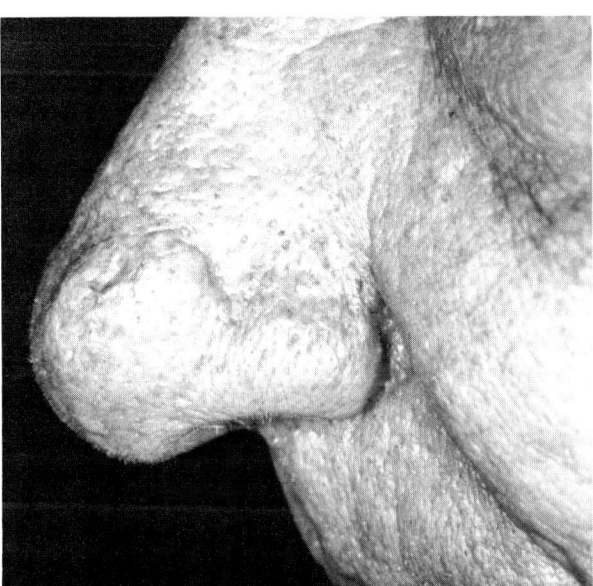

Figure 206. Focal area of rhinophyma of the nasal tip and ala preoperatively.

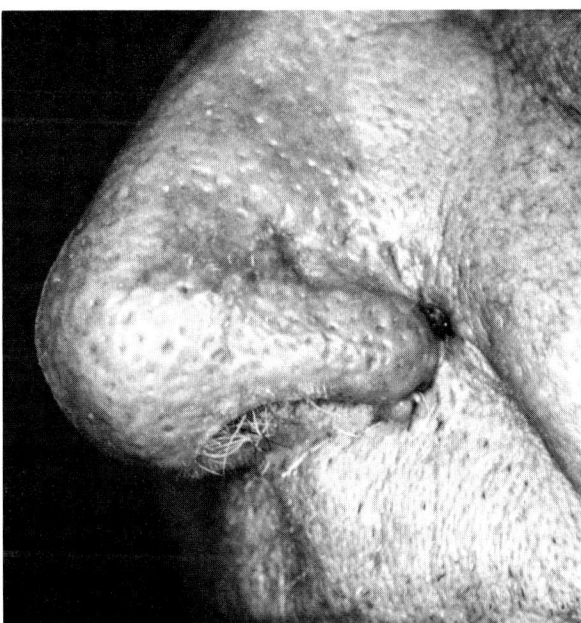

Figure 208. Cosmetic result six weeks postoperatively following localized area of treatment of the nasal tip and ala.

Figure 209. Bulbous enlargement of the nasal tip is seen in this frontal view preoperatively.

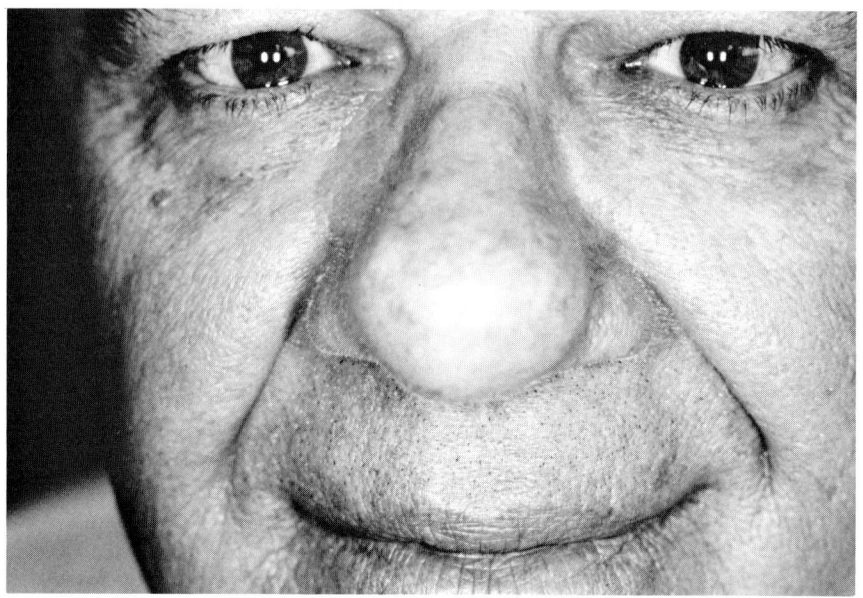

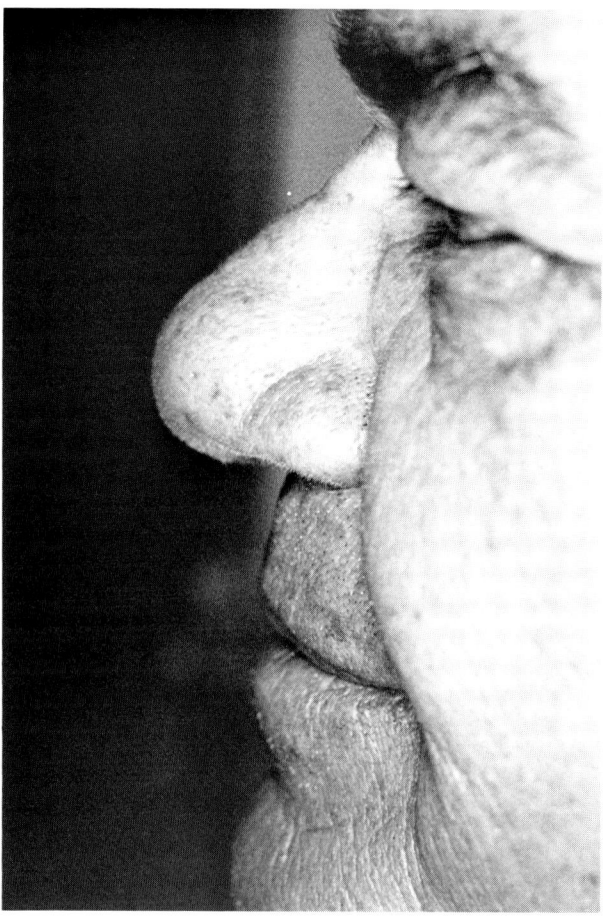

Figure 210. Enlargement of the nasal tip can also be seen laterally in this preoperative photograph.

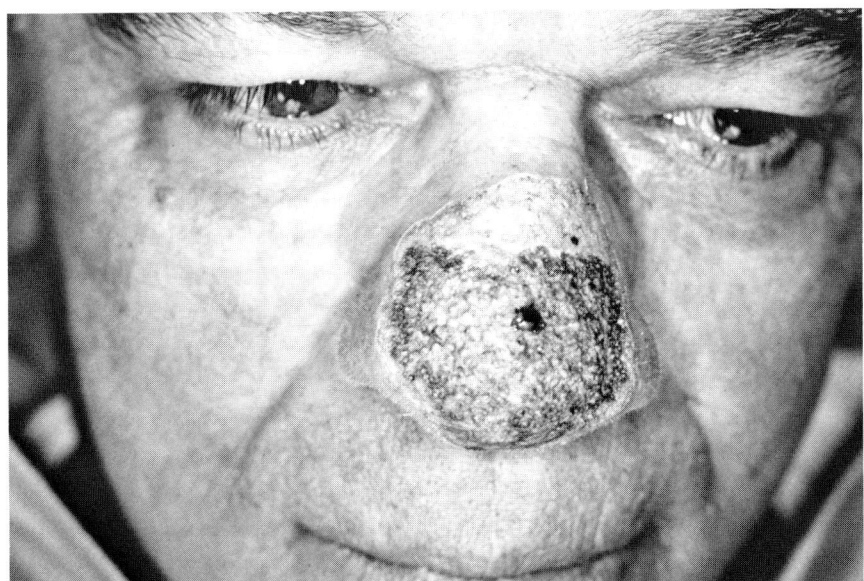

Figure 211. Only the area of hypertrophy has been vaporized in this frontal view seen immediately postoperatively.

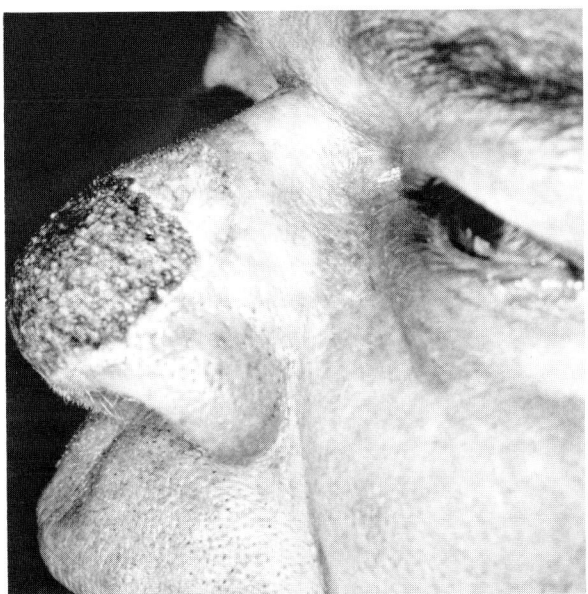

Figure 212. Lateral view demonstrates the localized area of treatment.

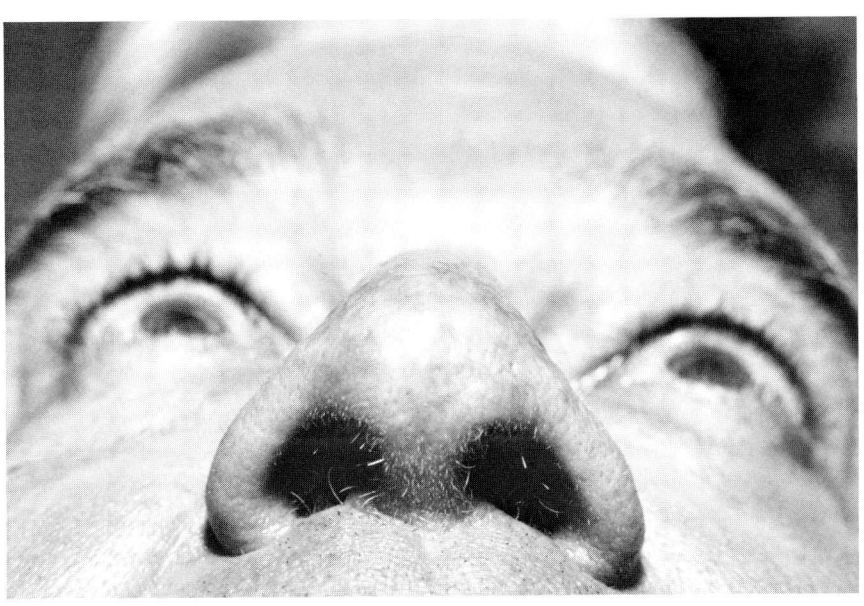

Figure 213. Clinical appearance five weeks postoperatively showing excellent cosmetic results and a decrease in the bulbous enlargement of the nasal tip of patient shown in Figures 209 and 210.

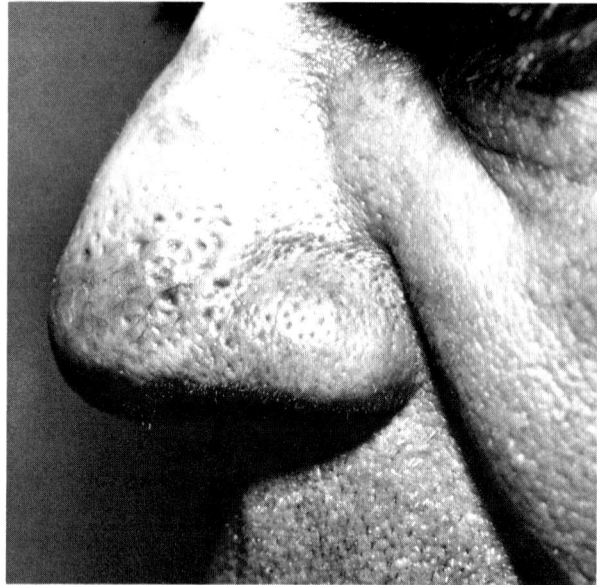

Figure 214. Lateral appearance of patient shown in Figure 210 six weeks postoperatively showing reduction in size and no adverse scarring.

the nasal skin may remain slightly red in color for an additional 3 to 6 weeks, the final textural results are usually superior to those obtained with other destructive techniques previously used in the treatment of this condition. Smaller degrees of nasal enlargement can also be treated (Figures 201 – 214) with good results.

BIBLIOGRAPHY

Apfelberg DB, Maser MR, Lash H, et al: Treatment of xanthelasma palpebrarum with the carbon dioxide laser. J Dermatol Surg Oncol 13:149–151, 1987.

Bailin PL, Ratz JL, Levine HL: Removal of tattoos by CO_2 laser. J Dermatol Surg Oncol 6:997–1001, 1980.

Bailin PL, Kantor GR, Wheeland RG: Carbon dioxide laser vaporization of lymphangioma circumscriptum. J Am Acad Dermatol 14:257–262, 1986.

Buecker JW, Ratz JL, Richfield DF: Histology of portwine stain treated with carbon dioxide laser. J Am Acad Dermatol 10:1014–1019, 1984.

Huerter CJ, Wheeland RG: Multiple eruptive vellus hair cysts treated with carbon dioxide (CO_2) laser vaporization. J Dermatol Surg Oncol 13:260–263, 1987.

Levine H, Bailin P: Carbon dioxide laser treatment of cutaneous hemangiomas and tattoos. Arch Otolaryngol 108:236–238, 1982.

McBurney E, Rosen D: Carbon dioxide laser treatment of verrucae vulgares. J Dermatol Surg Oncol 10:45–48, 1984.

Ratz JL, Bailin PL, Levin HL: CO_2 laser treatment of portwine stains: A preliminary report. J Dermatol Surg Oncol 8:1039–1044, 1982.

Ratz JL, Bailin PL, Wheeland RG: CO_2 laser treatment of epidermal nevi. J Dermatol Surg Oncol 12:567–570, 1986.

Roenigk RK, Ratz JL: CO_2 laser treatment of cutaneous neurofibromas. J Dermatol Surg Oncol 13:187–190, 1987.

Shapshay SM, Strong MS, Anastasi GW, et al: Removal of rhinophyma with the carbon dioxide laser: A preliminary report. Arch Otolaryngol 106:257–259, 1980.

Tan OT, Carney JM, Margolis R, et al: Histologic responses of portwine stains treated by argon, carbon dioxide and tunable dye lasers. A preliminary report. Arch Dermatol 122:1016–1022, 1986.

Wheeland RG, Ashley JR, Smith DA, et al: Carbon dioxide (CO_2) laser treatment of granuloma faciale. J Dermatol Surg Oncol 10:730–733, 1984.

Wheeland RG, Bailin PL, Kronberg E: Carbon dioxide (CO_2) laser vaporization for the treatment of multiple trichoepithelioma. J Dermatol Surg Oncol 10:470–475, 1984.

Wheeland RG, Bailin PL, Kantor GR, et al: Treatment of adenoma sebaceum with carbon dioxide laser vaporization. J Dermatol Surg Oncol 11:861–864, 1985.

Wheeland RG, Bailin PL, Reynolds OD, et al: Carbon dioxide (CO_2) laser vaporization of multiple facial syringomas. J Dermatol Surg Oncol 12:225–228, 1986.

Wheeland RG, Walker NPJ: Lasers — 25 years later. Internat J Dermatol 25:209–216, 1986.

5   Excisional Surgery Performed with the Carbon Dioxide Laser

In the excisional mode of operation (Table 8), the carbon dioxide laser is used with the laser beam focused to a small diameter of 0.1 to 0.2 mm. The power of the laser system is set to between 15 and 35 watts which yields an irradiance of between 50,000 and 100,000 W/cm². In this fashion, the carbon dioxide laser can function as a scalpel to incise soft tissue in relatively bloodless fashion (Table 9). The quality of hemostasis obtained with the laser as well as the speed with which the incision can be performed are both functions of the irradiance and the speed with which the laser surgeon moves the carbon dioxide laser beam along the incision line. The higher the irradiance and slower the beam is moved, the more rapidly the surgeon can proceed and the deeper the incision will be made.

The beginning laser surgeon should utilize a small stylus which is attached to the end of the laser handpiece to help determine the exact focal length of the laser that is being utilized. In this way, the beam of laser energy will not inadvertently become defocused and cause vaporization of the wound edges or base. The laser surgeon can, with practice, perform incisions with the carbon dioxide laser with the same skill as can be obtained with a scalpel. There is no doubt, however, that additional practice is required in order to obtain this degree of skill. While laser incisions cannot be performed, in general, as quickly as scalpel incisions, the length of the surgical procedure is usually no longer than the same procedure performed with a scalpel since additional time is not spent obtaining hemostasis, which is readily obtained as the carbon dioxide laser beam makes the incision.

In most cases, the laser will routinely seal blood vessels up to 0.5 mm in diameter along the incision line even in anticoagulated patients. If a low pressure blood vessel of greater size is encountered, routine hemostasis can even be obtained in that situation as well. For higher pressure vascular systems, the hemostatic properties of the laser may not be complete and some bleed-ing may, indeed, occur. If bleeding should occur from larger blood vessels, they can frequently be heat-sealed by grasping the end of the bleeding vessel with a pair of fine-tooth forceps and then, by defocusing the carbon dioxide laser beam, have their ends vaporized and welded shut with the carbon dioxide laser energy. It is prudent to always have electrocoagulative equipment available in the operating room in the event that vessels are encountered which cannot be sealed with the carbon dioxide laser.

Even though the quality of hemostasis obtained using the carbon dioxide laser for incisional or excisional surgery yields a totally dry wound, this does not prevent the laser surgeon from using skin flaps to repair a cutaneous wound. Also, closure of wounds with skin grafts, either full-thickness or split-thickness, can also be successful even if the dry defect was created with the laser. Of course, primary closure of a wound created by carbon dioxide laser excision is also not a problem, even though there is evidence that scalpel-incised wounds heal with greater tensile strength than similar laser-incised wounds, at least until three weeks postoperatively. Thereafter, the tensile strength of both wounds are identical. While this may be of concern to the beginnning laser surgeon, it does not appear to be of clinical relevance. The reason that this delay in tensile strength occurs may be due to the fact that the initial fibrin clot does not form following laser incision as it does with standard scalpel incision. As a consequence, all subsequent steps in the wound healing process are delayed. The final cosmetic result and the tensile strength of the wound remains unaltered whether the wound is created with the carbon dioxide laser or with a scalpel.

One tremendous advantage that the carbon dioxide laser lends the laser surgeon when performing excisional surgery is in undermining. Since the laser does not actually contact tissue, there is both minimal trauma to the soft tissue as well as increased ease of dissection. Undermin-

Table 8.   CO₂ Laser Excision

Power 15–35 watts
Irradiance 50,000–100,000 watts/cm²
Continuous mode
Focused 0.1–0.2 mm impact spot size (beam diameter)
Advantages
  Sterility
  Hemostasis—seals blood vessels up to 0.5 mm in
    diameter
  Lymphatics sealed to decrease postoperative swelling,
    and minimize metastasis by tumors
  Decreased postoperative pain by sealing of nerve endings
  Preservation of histology
  Minimal thermal injury to adjacent normal tissue
  No effect on pacemakers or other electronic monitoring
    equipment
  Will provide a relative bloodless field even in anticoag-
    ulated patients
Disadvantages
  Expense of equipment
  Bulky handpiece
  Vacuum system required
  Smoke and smell
  Safety precautions required

ing an inch or more beyond the incision line is not difficult for the skilled laser surgeon and there are fewer complications with hematoma formation that may occur if extensive undermining is done by blunt technique. Additionally, since the carbon dioxide laser also seals cutaneous lymphatic channels as it incises tissue, there may be at least a theoretic advantage in using the carbon dioxide laser in oncologic surgery. This may also explain the reason why there is less postoperative swelling when using the laser for

Table 9.   The Carbon Dioxide Laser

Excisional (focused) mode of operation
  Rhinophyma
  Keloids
    Lichen (acne) keloidalis nuchae
    Earlobe
  Bloodless surgery
    Highly vascular tissue (scalp)
    Anticoagulated patients
  Treatment of cutaneous malignancies
    Mohs surgery
    Excision of stromal independent neoplasms
      Squamous cell carcinoma
      Melanoma
      Carcinoma-in situ (Bowen's carcinoma)
      Dermatofibrosarcoma protuberans
    Perforation of exposed cranial bone
    Patients with pacemakers that restrict electrosurgical
      instrumentation

incisional surgery. Likewise, since the laser will also seal the small sensory nerve endings of the skin, postoperative discomfort with laser surgery is frequently minimal.

Another advantage in performing laser excisional surgery is the fact that laser energy does not interfere with pacemakers or operating room monitors. When using electrosurgical instrumentation, interference may occur with these monitors. Additionally, some pacemakers can be readjusted if certain types of electrosurgical apparatus are utilized instead of the laser.

Since the laser can be focused to a minute beam, its delivery to tissue can be extremely fine. Likewise, since carbon dioxide laser energy is absorbed by intracellular and extracellular water, there is minimal thermal injury to the surrounding normal skin. These two factors permit tissue removed with the laser to be examined histologically without significant loss of detail. This compares strikingly to the histologic appearance of tissue that has been removed with some electrosurgical instruments.

TECHNIQUE FOR PERFORMING LASER INCISIONAL SURGERY

While there are no substantial differences in laser incisional surgical techniques compared to that required for scalpel incisions, several changes are required. First, the wound must not be prepared with a flammable, antiseptic agent like isopropyl alcohol. Secondly, the sterile surgical drapes must either be nonflammable or moistened with sterile saline or sterile water to prevent accidental ignition through inadvertent contact with the carbon dioxide laser beam. Third, the patient and all operating room personnel must wear protective eyeglasses or goggles to limit the potential for inadvertent injury to the eyes. Fourth, a smoke evacuator designed especially for carbon dioxide laser surgery must be utilized to remove the noxious gases and steam from the operating room. The nozzle of the smoke evacuator tubing and the laser handpiece must be sterilized. If the carbon dioxide laser arm must extend over the operative field, this must also be covered with a sterile sleeve to prevent inadvertent contamination of the surgical site. Once these minor modifications have been made, no further variations are required from the standard excisional surgical technique.

Once the incision or excision has been performed and the wound is ready for repair, it is important to check the incision line to be sure that there has been no inadvertent vaporization along the depth of the incision margin. If vaporization accidentally occurs, it results in the formation of a small deposit of carbonized particles or char. If this char is left in the incision line it will appear as a small brown line after the wound heals. Furthermore, it may delay wound healing since this material must be removed by cellular phagocytosis. As a consequence, it is quite easy to remove these small amounts of carbonized material with light scrubbing using a cotton-tipped applicator that has been soaked in sterile saline. If this pigment is not removed prior to closure, the surgeon can expect spontaneous improvement over a six to eight-week period of time.

EXCISION OF MALIGNANT MELANOMA

As an example of the quality of hemostasis and wound healing, a clinical example of excisional surgery of a malignant melanoma on the temple (Figures 215 and 216) will be described and illustrated. After the area of excision is first marked (Figure 217) using a sterile surgical marker, local anesthesia (Figure 218) is obtained. One-percent plain lidocaine can be utilized in this situation since hemostasis is so complete. A small "M-plasty" is created medially to shorten the length of the wound and more closely approximate the natural creases in this location (Figure 219).

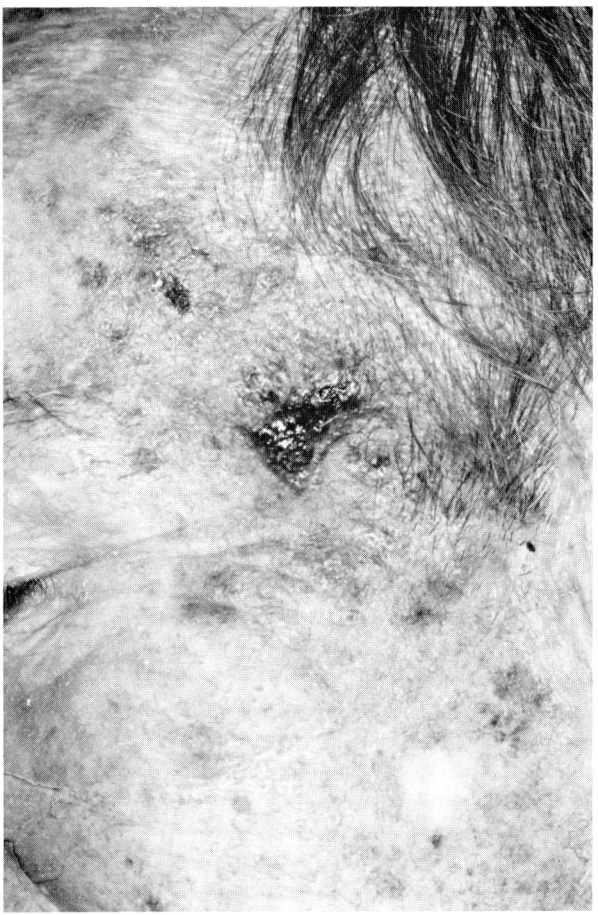

Figure 216. Appearance of same wound after biopsy has demonstrated malignant melanoma.

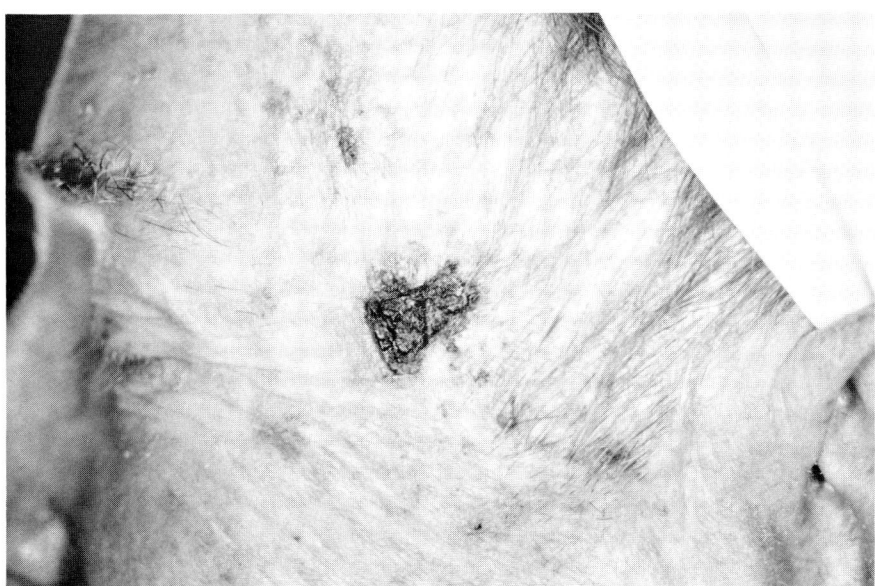

Figure 215. Initial appearance of a crusted lesion of the left temple. (See Figures 216–229.)

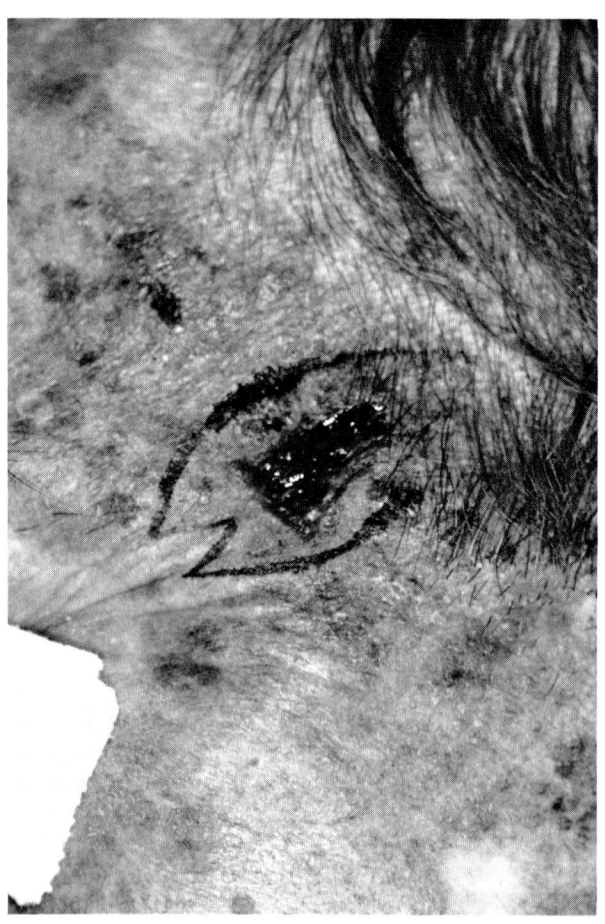

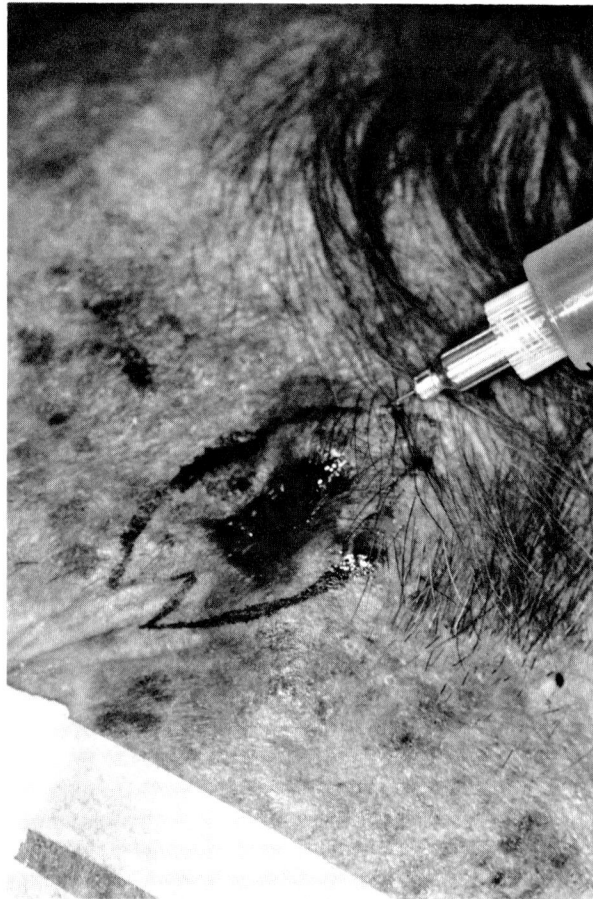

Figure 217.   A surgical marker outlines the planned excision.

Figure 218.   Injection of local anesthesia is performed.

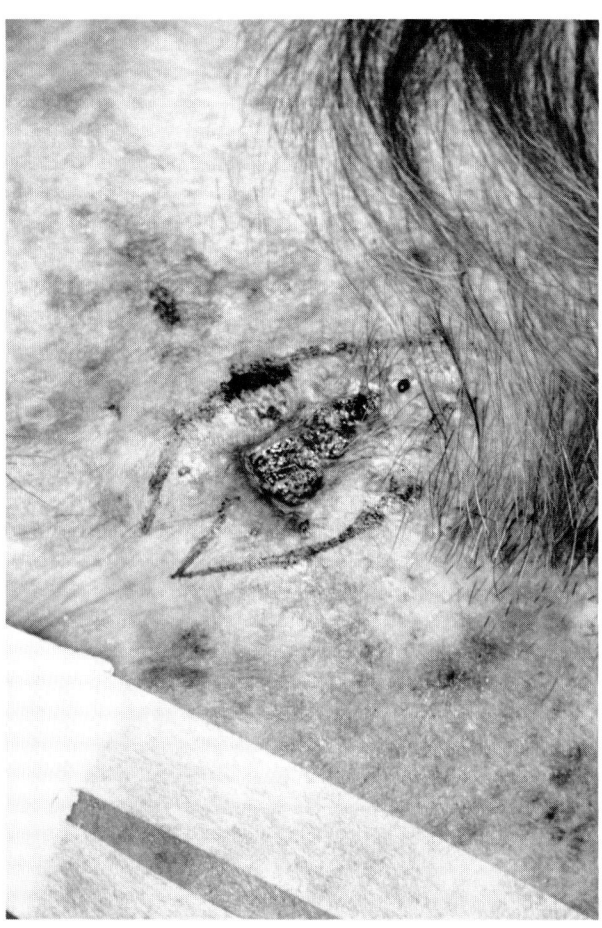

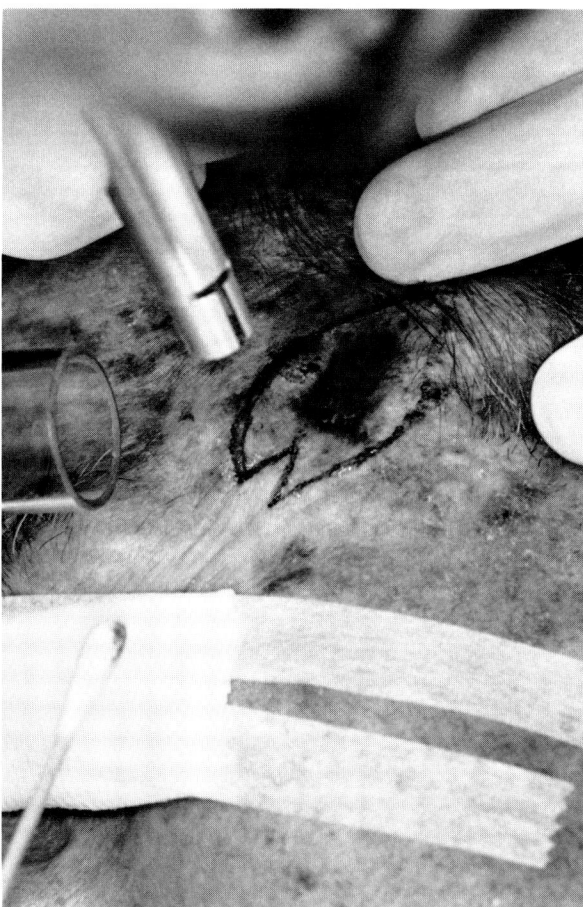

Figure 219. M-plasty shortens the length of the planned excision on the medial edge.

Figure 220. Using the focused carbon dioxide laser beam, the incision is begun at the superior edge.

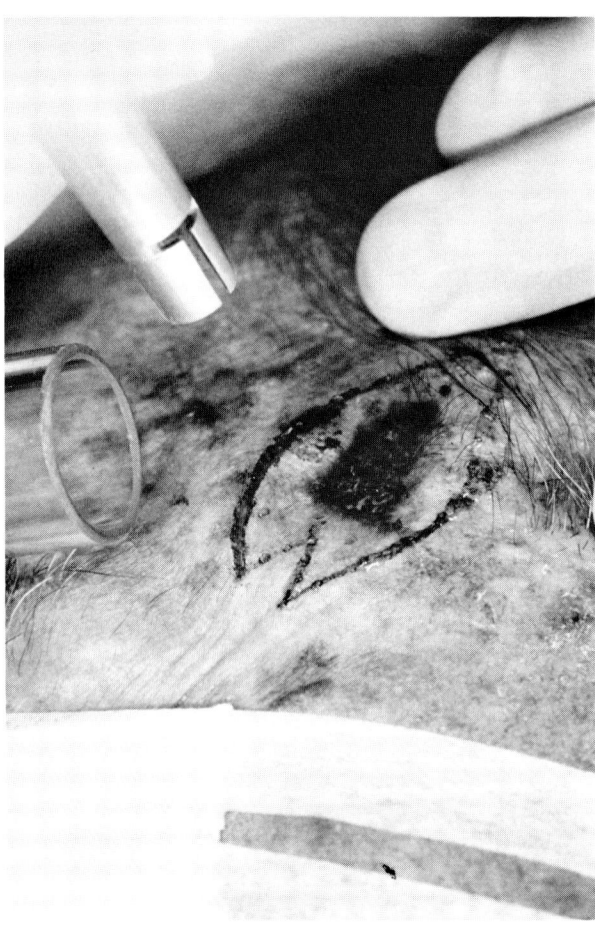

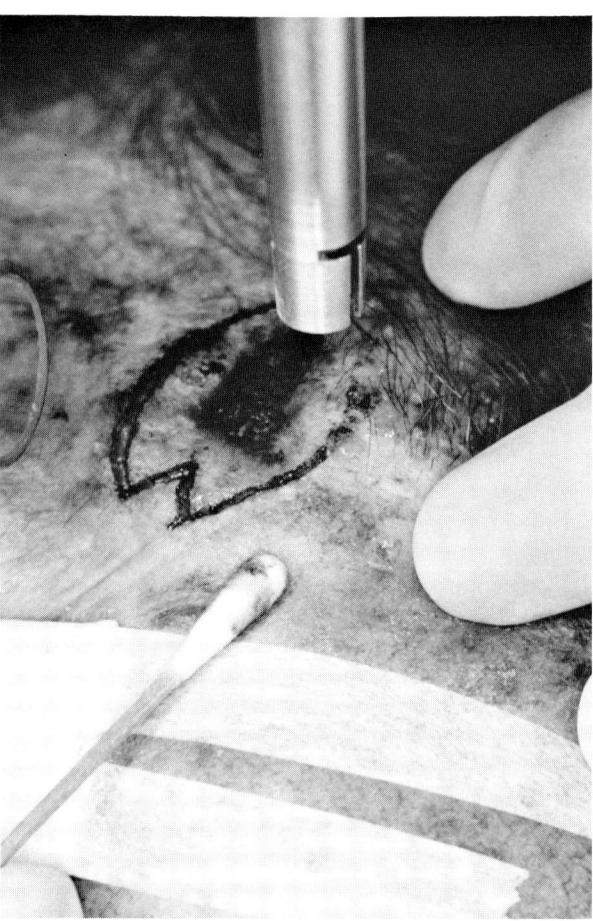

Figure 221. The helium-neon aiming beam, used for precise positioning of the carbon dioxide laser, can be seen at one end of the M-plasty.

Figure 222. The incision is continued around the inferior margin.

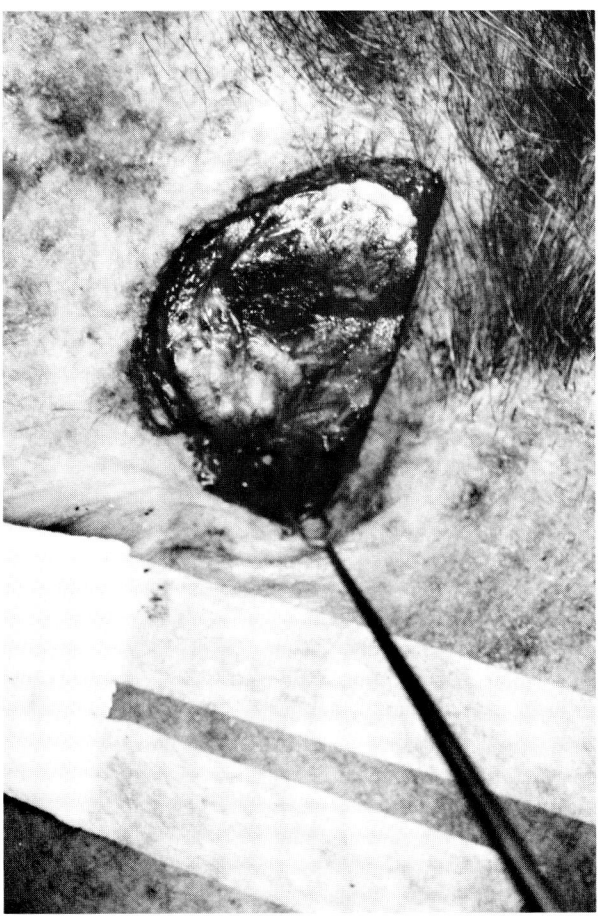 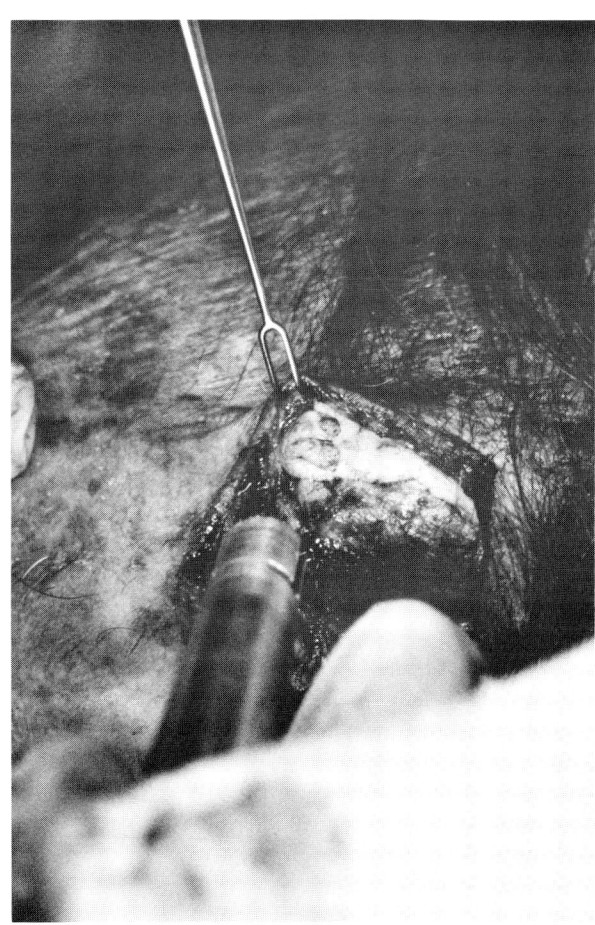

Figure 231. Additional undermining is performed using the carbon dioxide laser.

Figure 232. The superior edge of the wound is undermined in a similar fashion.

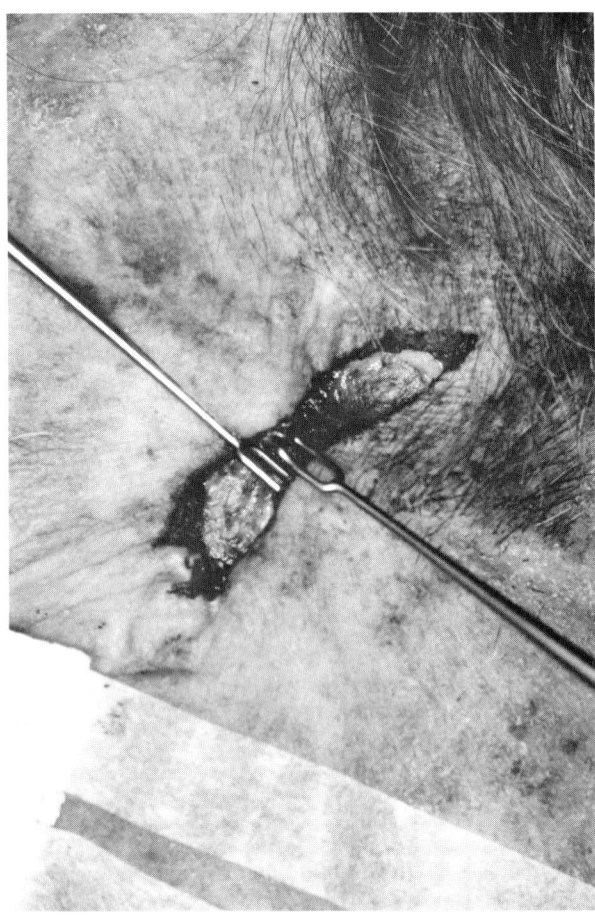

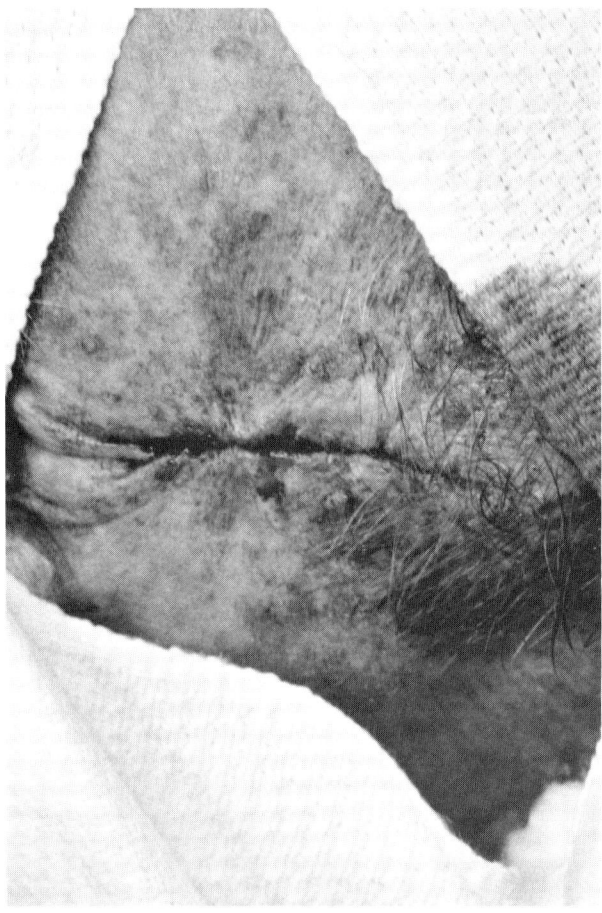

Figure 233.   The wound is tested for ease of closure with skin hooks.

Figure 234.   Appearance of the wound after placement of one buried subcuticular suture.

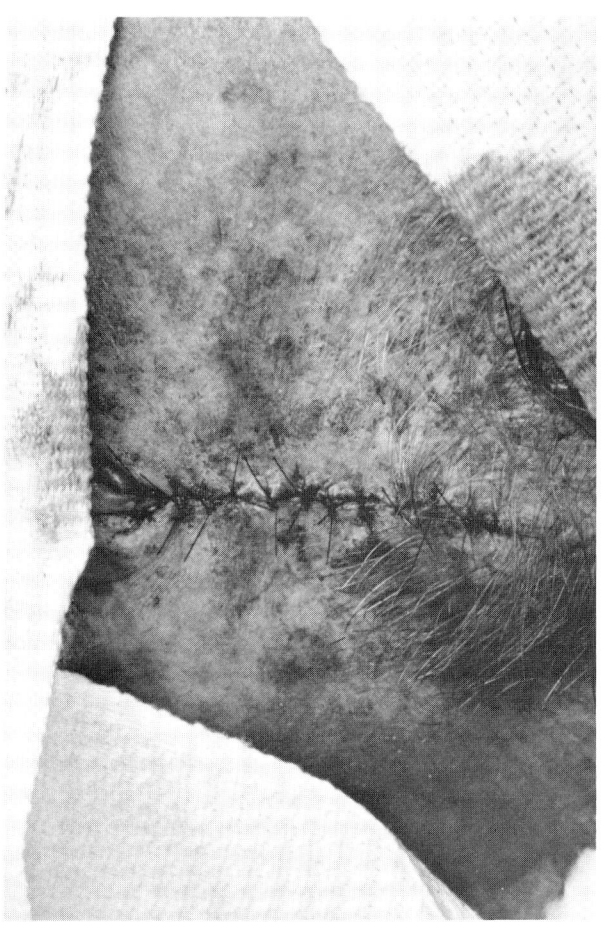

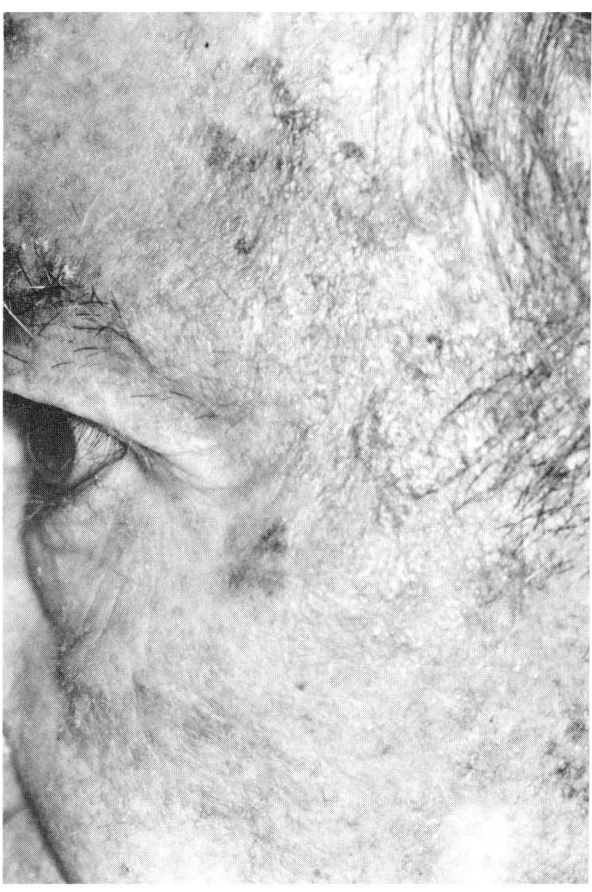

Figure 237. Final appearance of the wound six weeks postoperatively with an inconspicuous surgical scar.

Figure 235. Appearance of the wound immediately postoperatively with epidermal sutures in place.

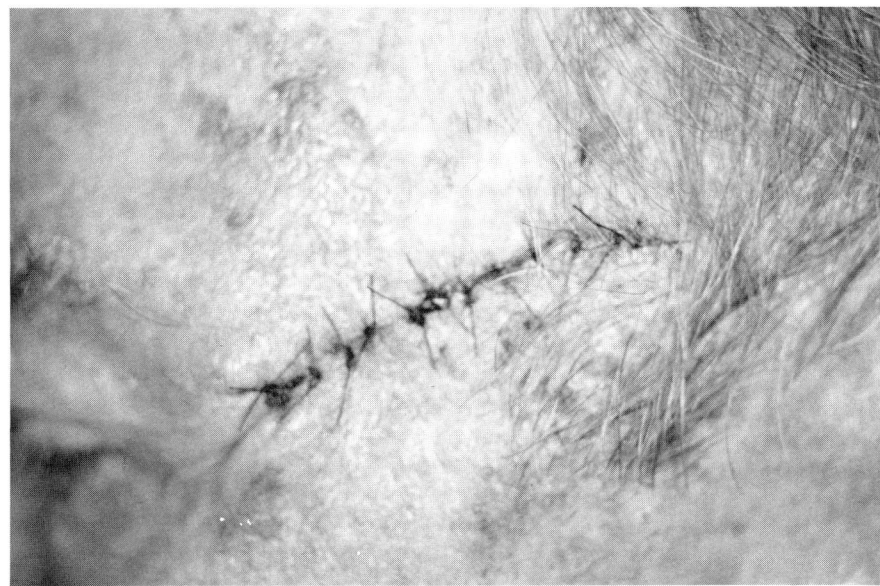

Figure 236. Clinical appearance of wound showing minimal thermal effect at time of suture removal nine days postoperatively.

The specimen can be interpreted completely by the pathologist due to minimal thermal effect caused by the focused carbon dioxide laser beam. This same incisional technique can be utilized for any of the stromal independent tumors such as melanoma or squamous cell carcinomas since the sealing of lymphatics lends, at least theoretically, an advantage to the patient by reducing the small chance of dissemination of malignant cells caused by manipulation occuring at the time of surgical intervention. In addition to being able to perform laser excision in patients with pacemakers or those patients who are being monitored during a surgical procedure, the carbon dioxide laser can also be used successfully in the excision of lesions in anticoagulated patients.

SCALP SURGERY WITH THE CARBON DIOXIDE LASER

Since the scalp is a very vascular tissue, the carbon dioxide laser has been employed in this location for a variety of different lesions. In treatment of male-pattern alopecia, a surgical procedure used to minimize the extent of balding on the crown of the head is known as scalp reduction. The carbon dioxide laser can be substituted for the scalpel in this procedure and bald tissue can be harvested with the focused carbon dioxide laser beam (Figures 238–246). Wound healing

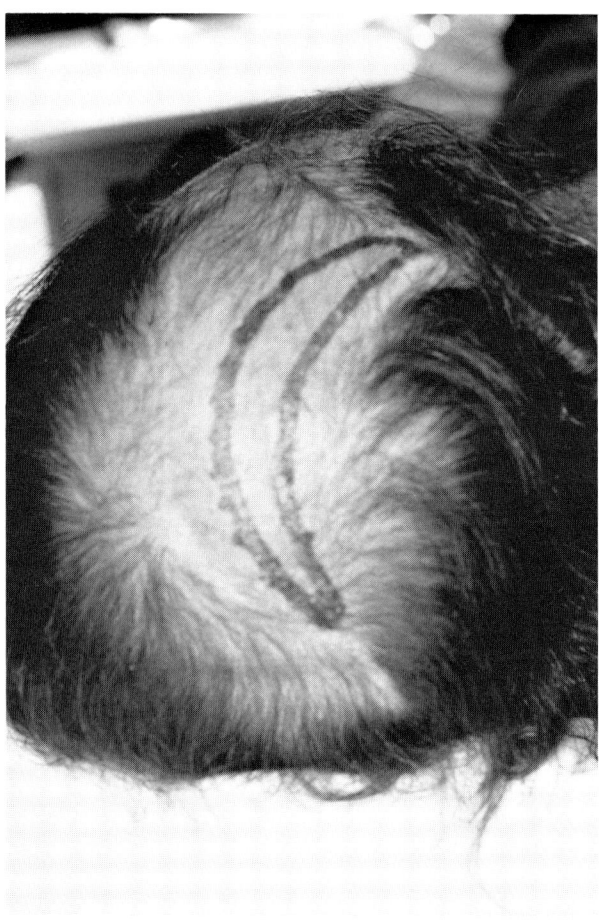

Figure 238. The planned excisional specimen for reduction of male-pattern baldness is outlined. (See Figures 239–247.)

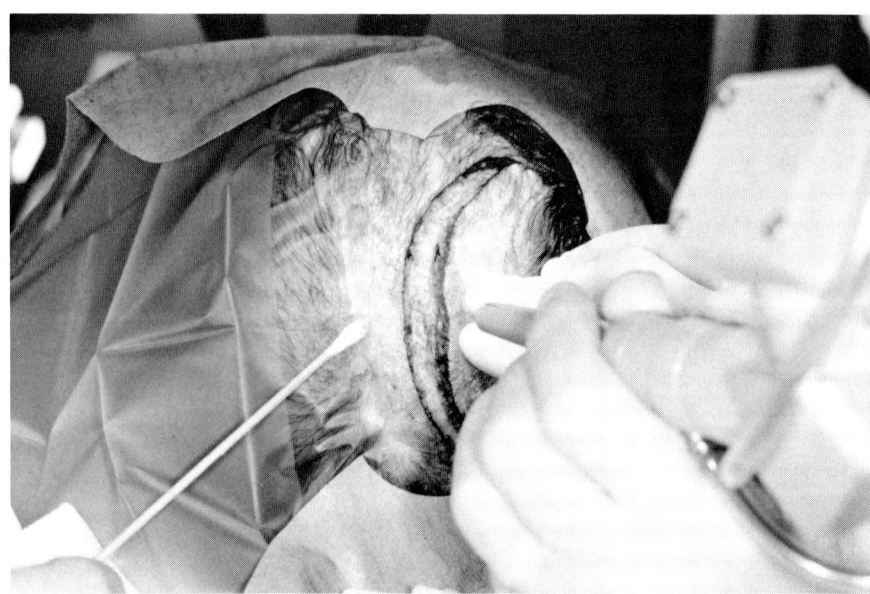

Figure 239. One side of the excisional specimen has been performed with the carbon dioxide laser in bloodless fashion.

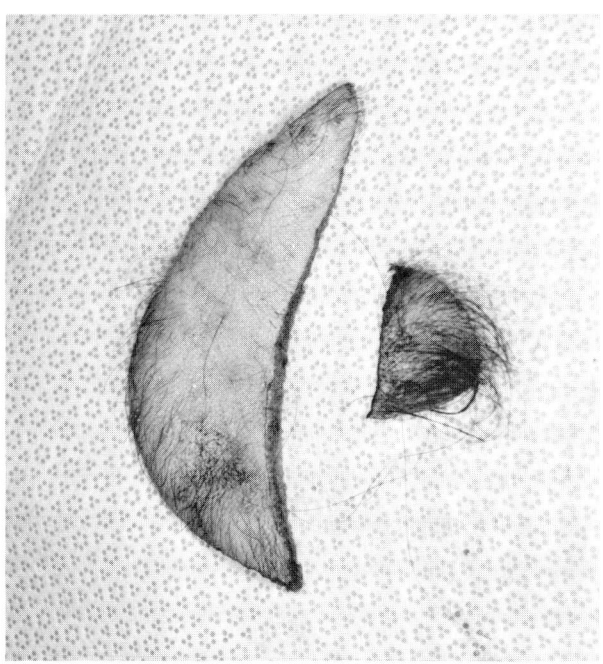

Figure 240. The appearance of the excisional specimen is seen.

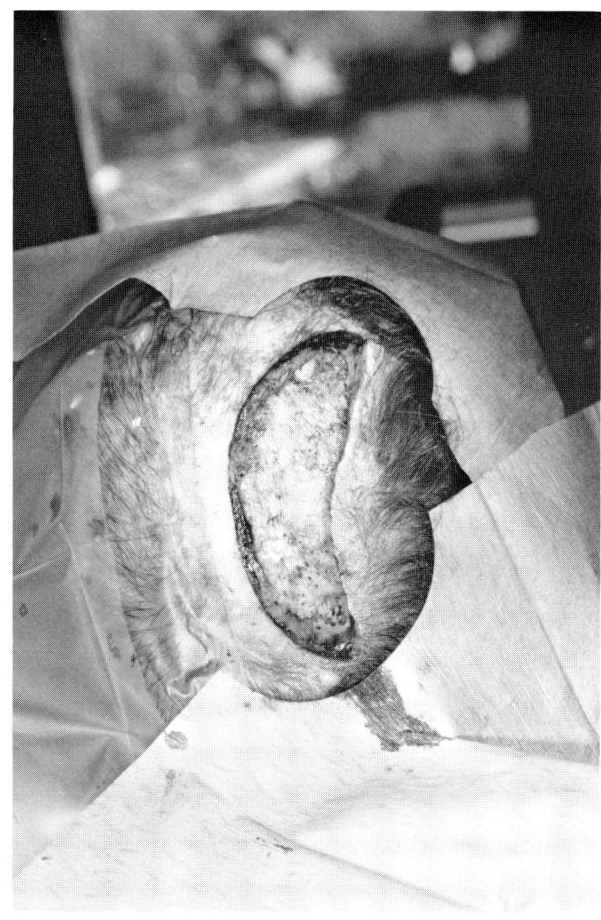

Figure 241. The final defect after carbon dioxide laser excision shows a bloodless surgical field.

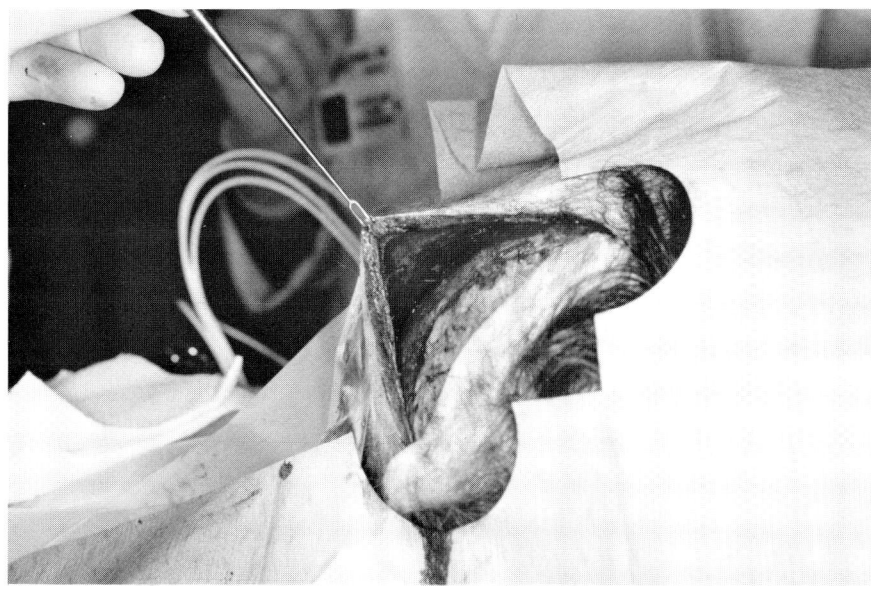

Figure 242. Undermining can be performed in this location with the laser.

Figure 243. The opposite side of the wound is now being undermined with the focused carbon dioxide laser.

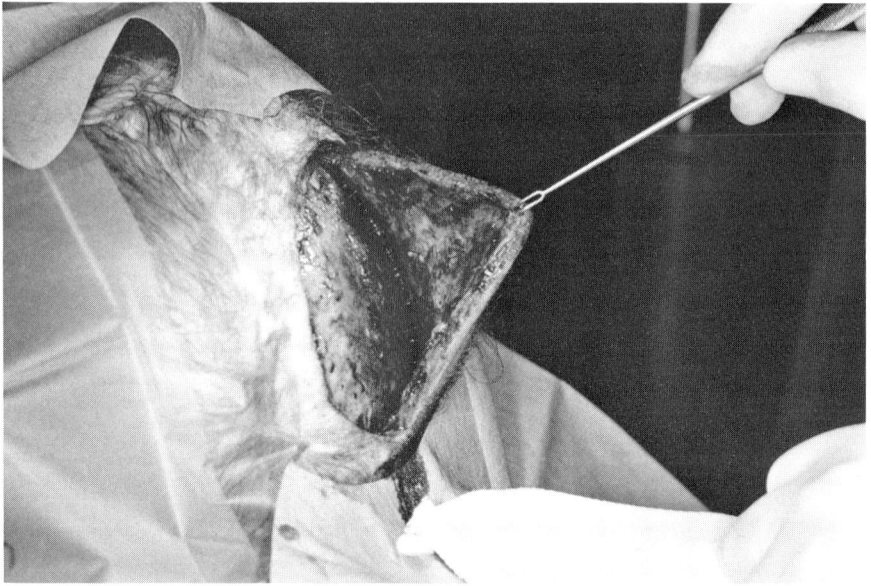

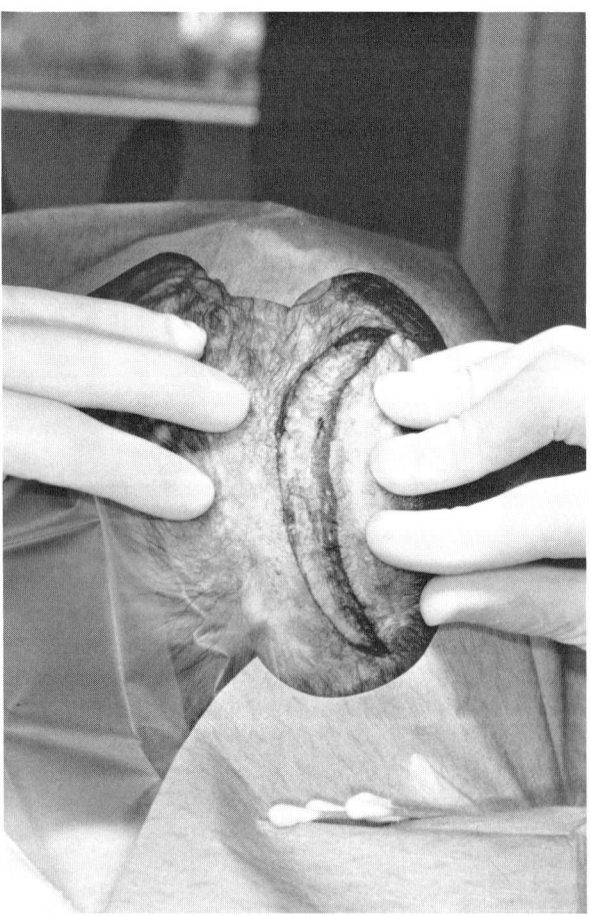

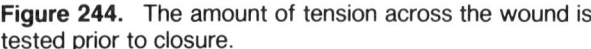

Figure 244. The amount of tension across the wound is tested prior to closure.

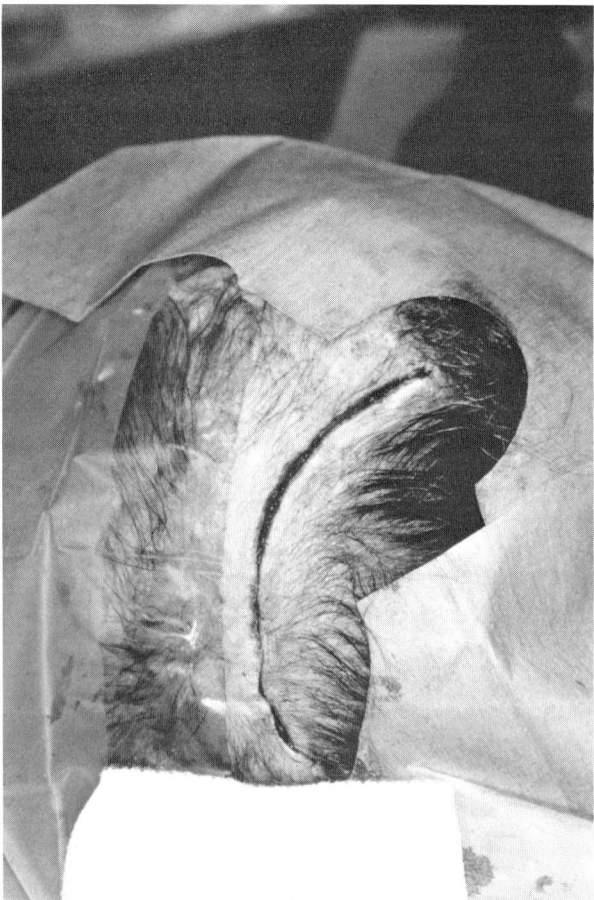

Figure 245. The appearance of the wound after placement of several subgaleal sutures.

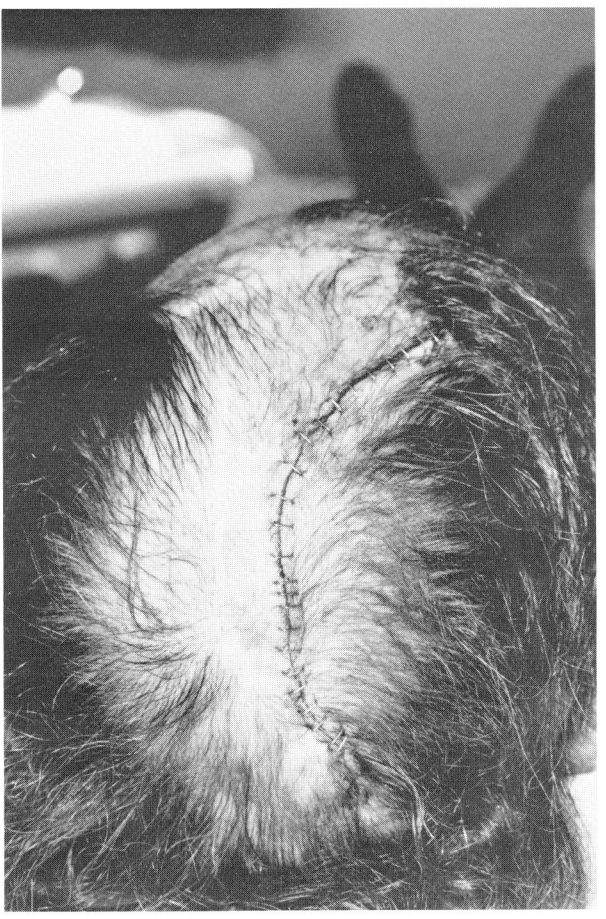

Figure 246. The appearance of the wound immediately postoperatively following closure with surgical staples.

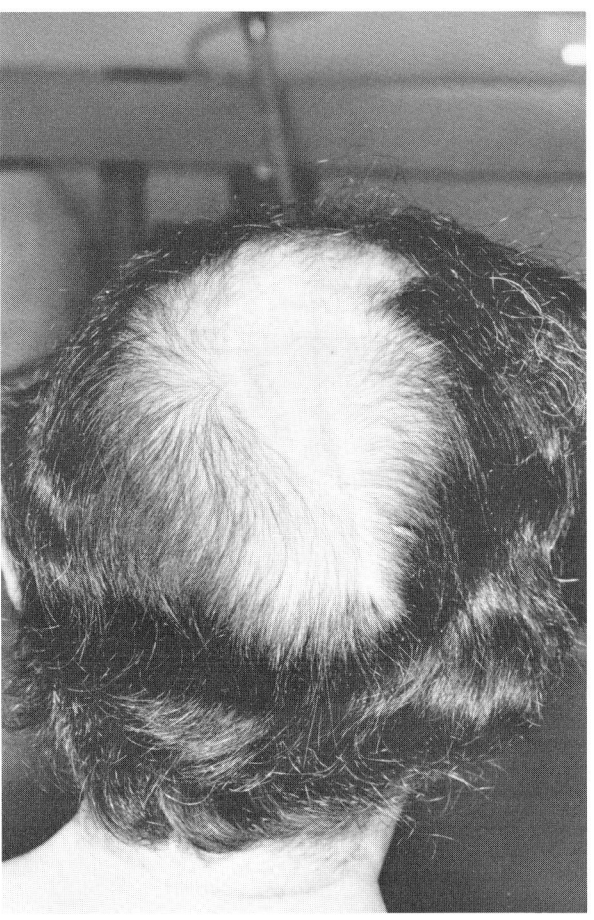

Figure 247. Final appearance of the wound three months postoperatively showing a relatively fineline surgical scar.

proceeds uneventfully (Figure 247). The quality of hemostasis obtained on the scalp helps the laser surgeon minimize blood loss.

LASER EXCISION OF KELOIDS AND ACNE KELOIDALIS NUCHAE

The carbon dioxide laser has proven to be extremely useful in the treatment of keloids of the head and neck. The reasons that carbon dioxide laser excisional surgery may be beneficial in these cases probably relates to the fact that the laser causes minimal trauma to surrounding tissue and, thus, the stimulus for the development of recurrent fibrosis and keloid are kept to an absolute minimum. The technique that is utilized in the treatment of keloids on the head and neck will be discussed.

Earlobe Keloids

Keloids of the ear may occur in any racial group, at any age, and from a variety of injuries; however, most keloids of the earlobe are secondary to ear piercing with presumed secondary infection of the epithelialized channel through the lobe. In the treatment of this condition, the patient must first be evaluated to determine whether the keloid is found on one aspect or the other of the lobe or if it completely penetrates through the ear lobe itself. If the keloid seems to be confined either to the anterior or posterior aspect of the lobe itself, then only that portion of the ear is treated. If, however, there is translobular involvement on palpation, the entire keloidal tract and the extensions on either end must be removed as a dumbbell in order to affect a cure (Figures 248 and 249).

Figure 248. A small keloidal papule is seen on the anterior surface of the left ear.

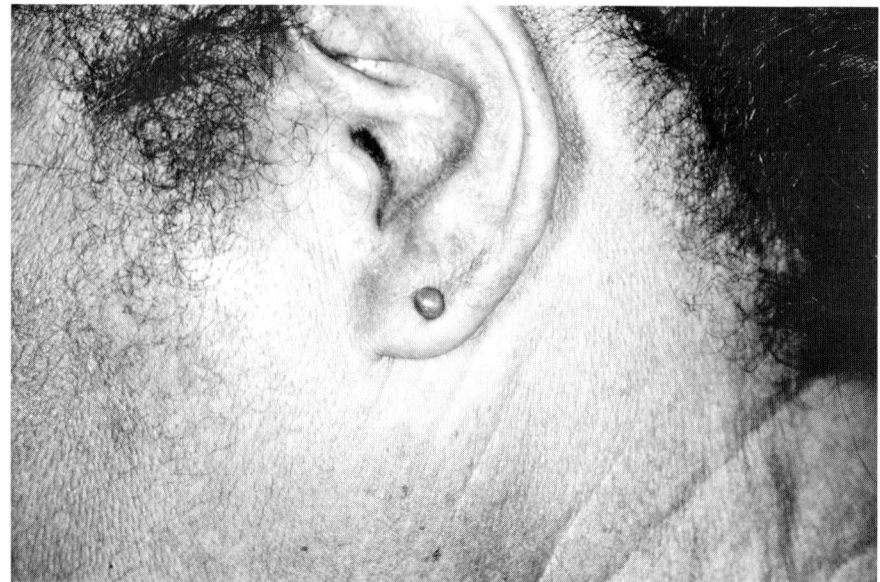

In this condition, local anesthesia is obtained. The portion of the keloid that is visible or palpable is excised using the carbon dioxide laser in its focused mode of operation. In general, the parameters used are a beam size of 0.1 mm, a power setting of 15 to 20 watts, and a continuous discharge mode. The keloid and the adjacent fibrotic soft tissue are excised using the focused mode of operation. If a through-and-through defect results (Figure 250), the anterior surface may be left to heal on its own or may be closed primarily with suture material (Figure 251). The posterior surface of a through-and-through defect is always allowed to granulate and heal by second intention (Figures 252 and 253). This serves to minimize tension across the healing wound which may be responsible for causing the reformation of a new keloid.

If, on the other hand, the keloid seems to be confined to only one aspect of the lobe (Figure 254), this tissue is shaved flush with the skin surrounding it using the focused carbon dioxide laser beam and the same parameters described above (Figure 255). In both cases after comple-

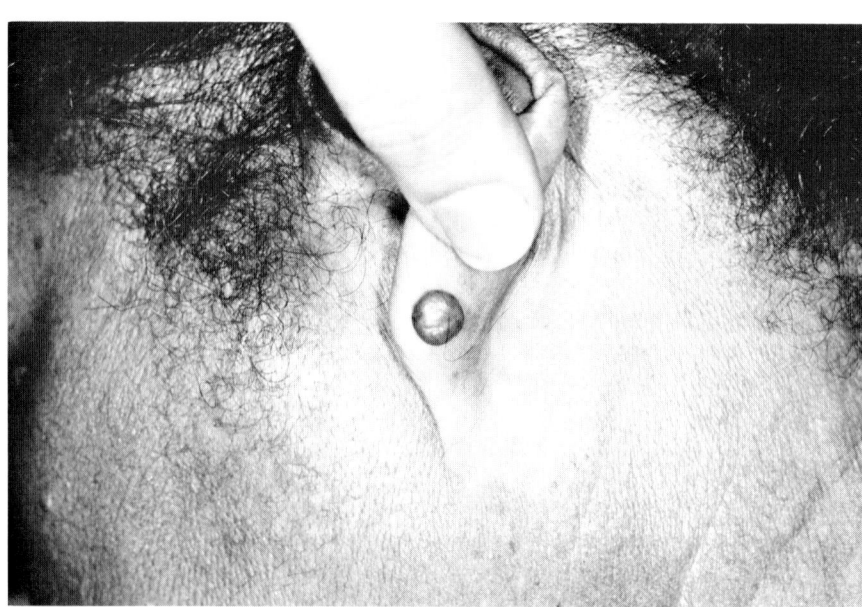

Figure 249. The keloid is also evident on the posterior aspect of the ear on the patient shown in Figure 248.

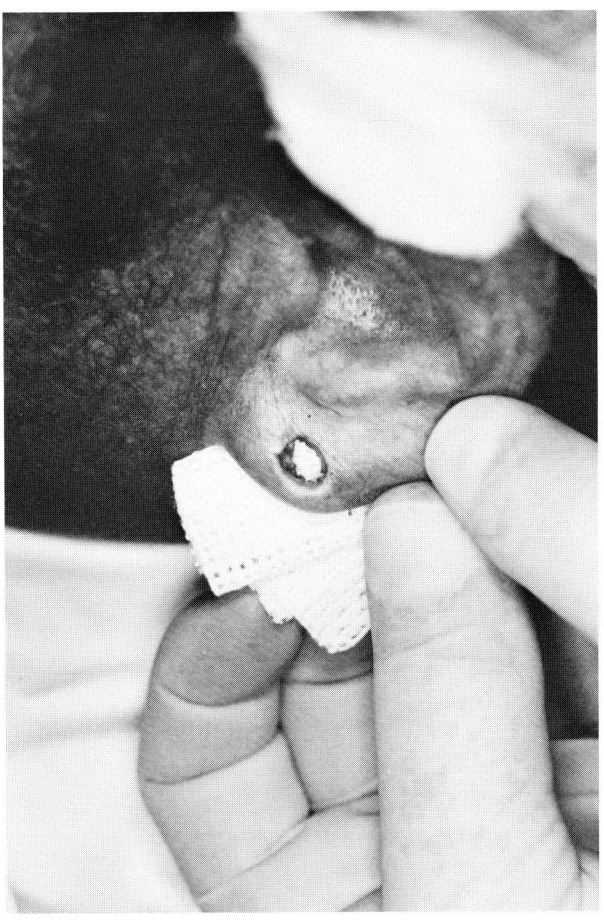

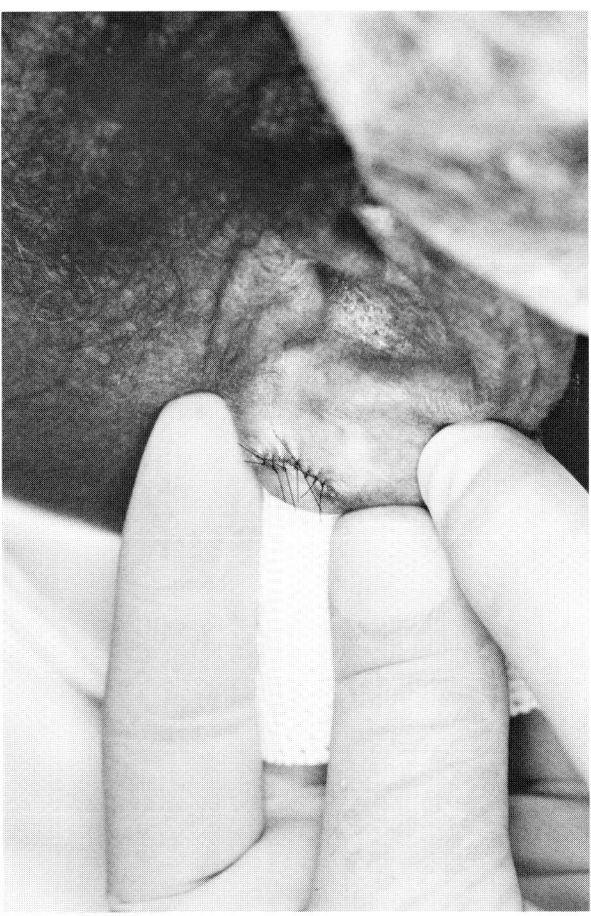

Figure 250. A through-and-through defect has resulted from carbon dioxide laser excision of this translobular keloid. (See Figures 251–253.)

Figure 251. The anterior surface of the wound has been repaired primarily.

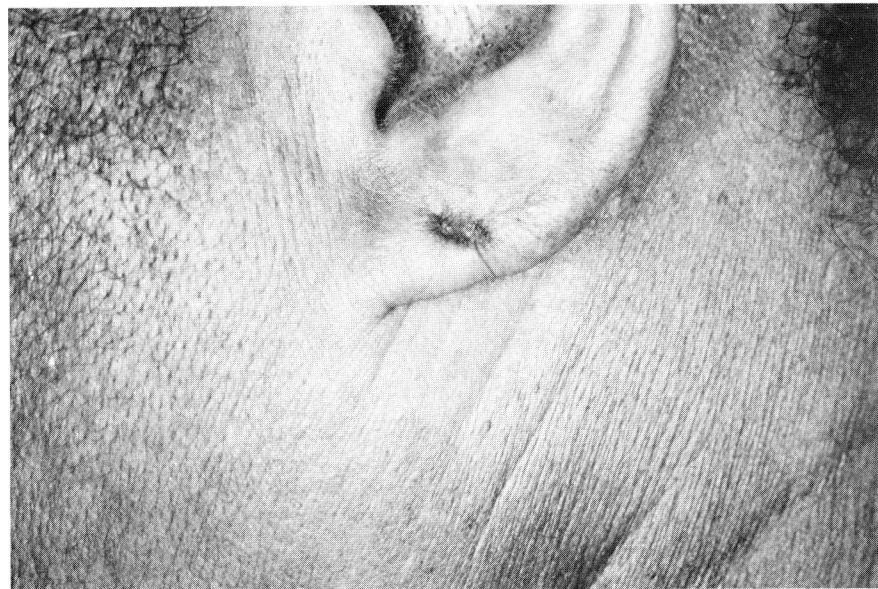

Figure 252. Postinflammatory hyperpigmentation is seen on the anterior surface of the ear four weeks postoperatively.

Figure 253. The posterior aspect of the ear, which has been allowed to heal by secondary intention, is seen four weeks postoperatively as a soft, flat, slightly hyperpigmented scar.

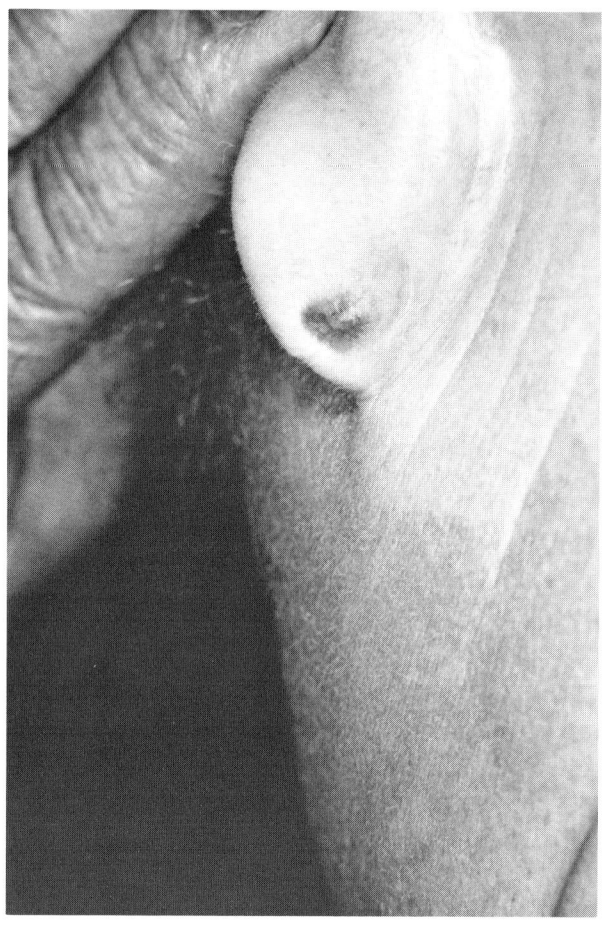

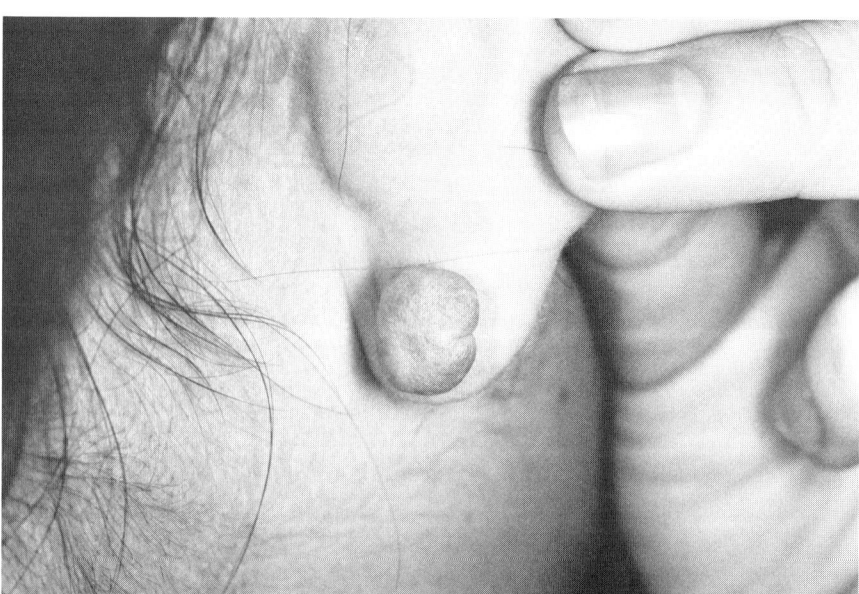

Figure 254. This keloid of the earlobe is confined to the posterior aspect of the lobe. (See Figures 255 and 256.)

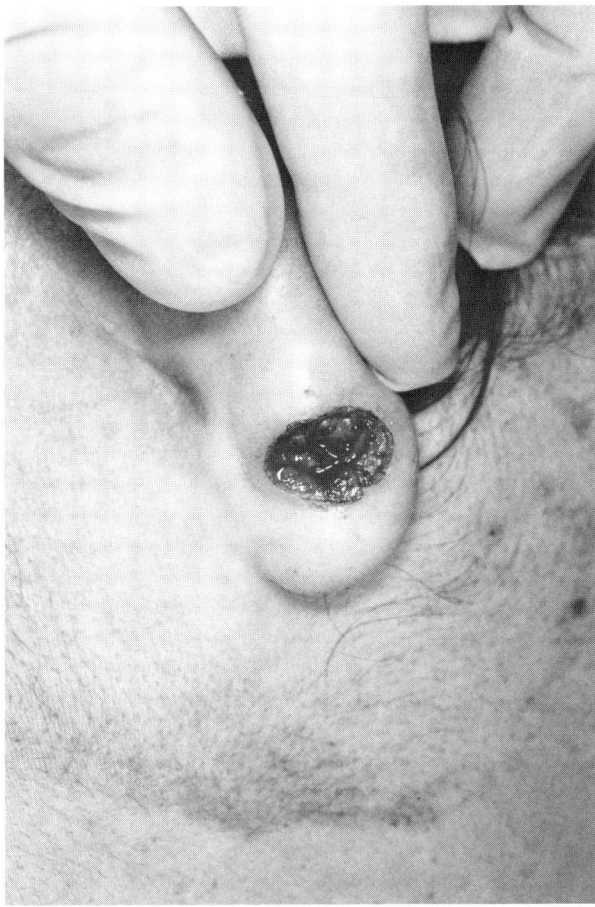

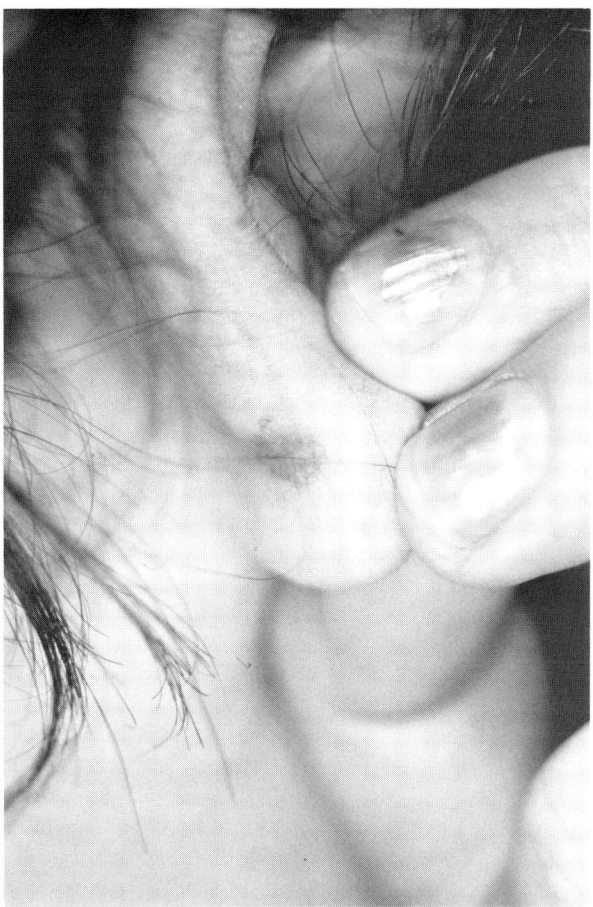

Figure 255. Following shave removal of the keloid with the carbon dioxide laser, a superficial defect is seen.

Figure 256. Six weeks after laser removal, the wound has healed by second intention with a good cosmetic result and a soft, flat scar.

tion of excision of the palpable or visible keloidal mass, the base of the wound is carefully examined and palpated to see if additional fibrotic material is present. Any persistent areas of fibrosis are subsequently removed using the focused laser beam. This process is continued layer by layer until no palpable fibrotic material is present.

If the keloid has recurred after previous therapy or if the surgeon is concerned about the subsequent development of a new keloid, the base and edges of the incised tissue are injected once with intralesional triamcinolone 40 mg/cc usually in a dose of 0.1 to 0.3 cc. The wound is then dressed in sterile fashion. Wound care consists of twice daily cleansing with hydrogen peroxide and application of an antibacterial ointment. The wound is allowed to heal by second intention which, depending upon size of the wound, usually is complete in three to six weeks (Figure 256).

Lichen Keloidalis Nuchae

This keloidal mass is typically found on the nape of the neck and results from the ingrowth of curly hairs into the skin of the scalp. The foreign body reaction that follows causes the development of fibrosis and keloidal scarring (Figure 257). This extremely difficult lesion to treat has been successfully managed with the carbon dioxide laser. The area of involvement is carefully examined and palpated for the extent of the lesion. This is then marked with a surgical marker and local anesthesia is obtained using 1% lidocaine. Using the focused laser, with a beam diameter of 0.1 mm, 20 watts of power and continuous discharge, this tissue is excised (Figure 258). The depth to which the excision is carried is dependent upon the level of fibrosis. After the mass of the keloid has been removed, the walls and base of the wound itself are carefully inspected and palpated for residual areas of fibrosis. If any

Figure 257. A large keloidal mass is seen preoperatively on the nape of the neck due to lichen keloidalis nuchae. (See Figures 258–262.)

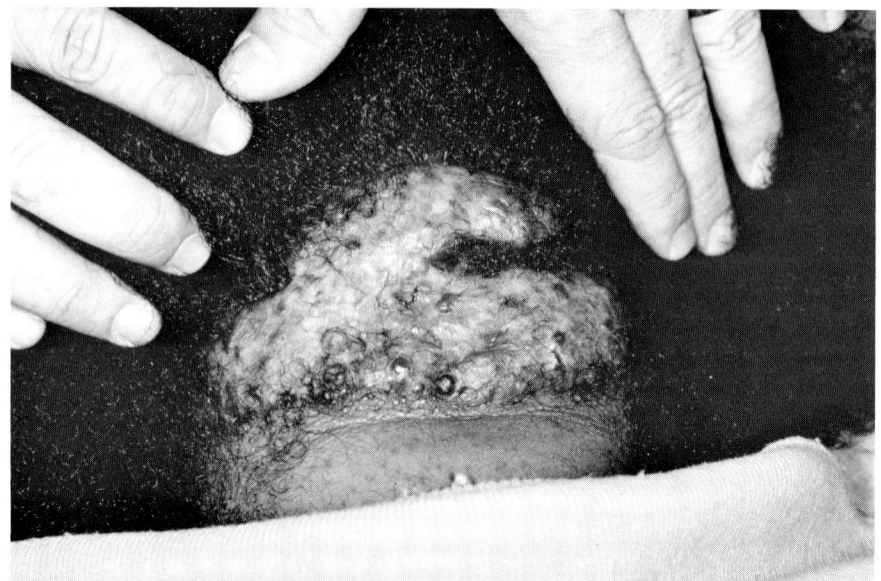

Figure 258. Using the focused carbon dioxide laser beam, the keloidal mass and all associated fibrotic material has been excised. *Note:* Focal areas of charring appear where persistent bleeding from small blood vessels occurred and was controlled with delivery of brief pulses of defocused carbon dioxide laser energy.

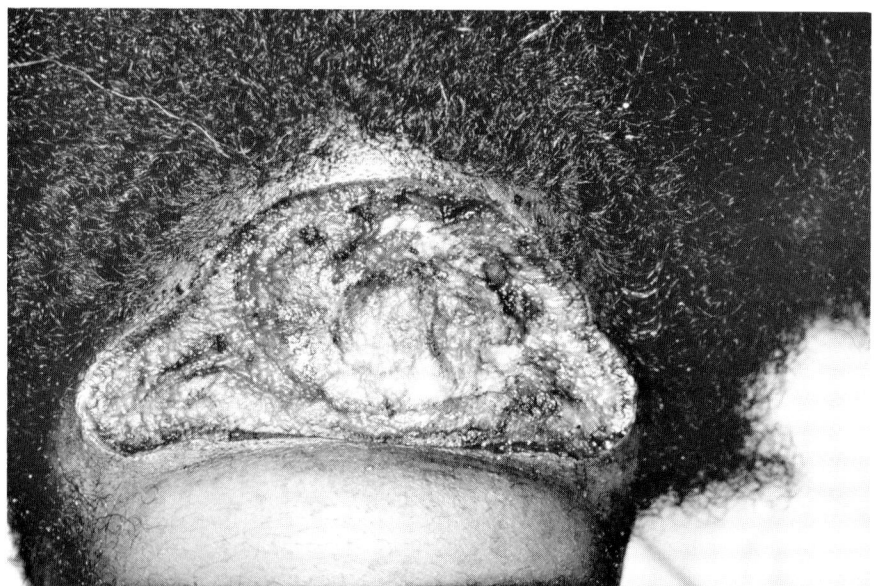

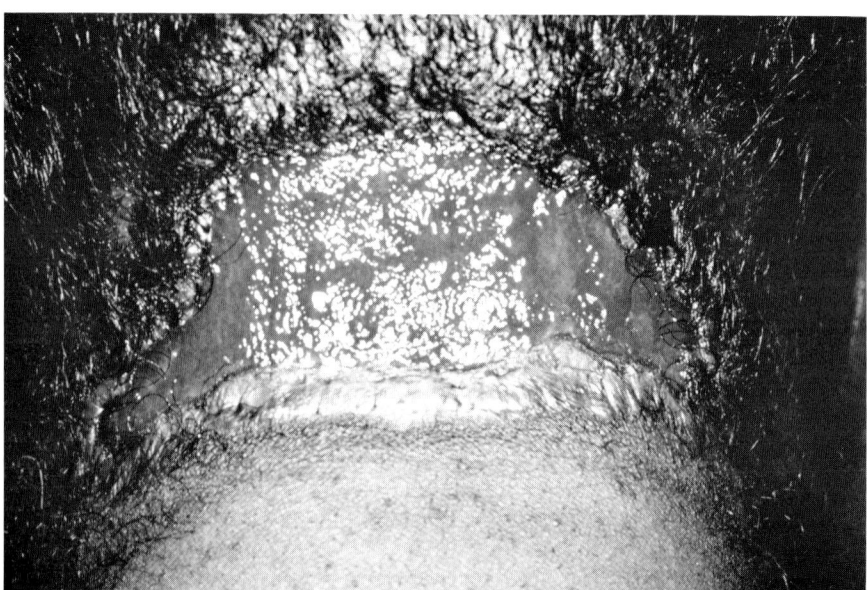

Figure 259. A clean granulating wound is present at four weeks postoperatively.

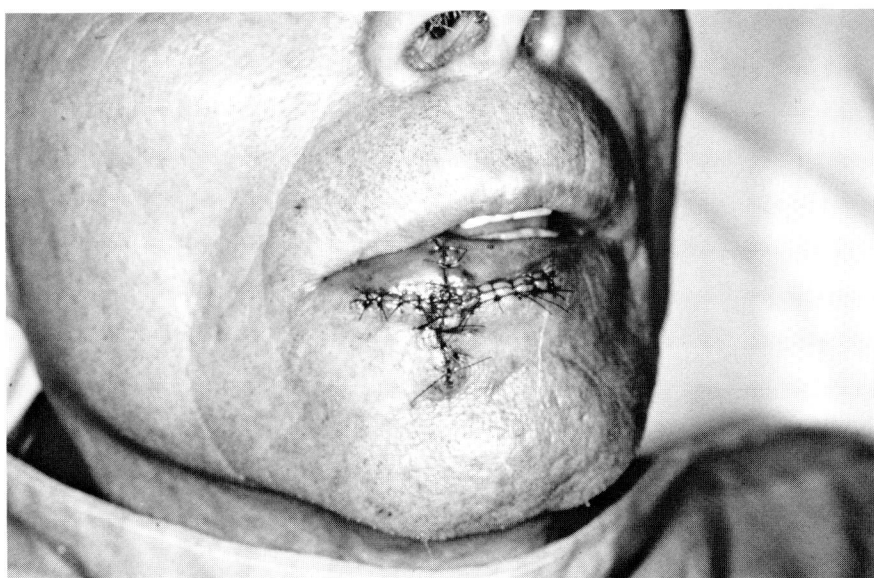

Figure 269. Final appearance of the patient following immediate repair of this defect.

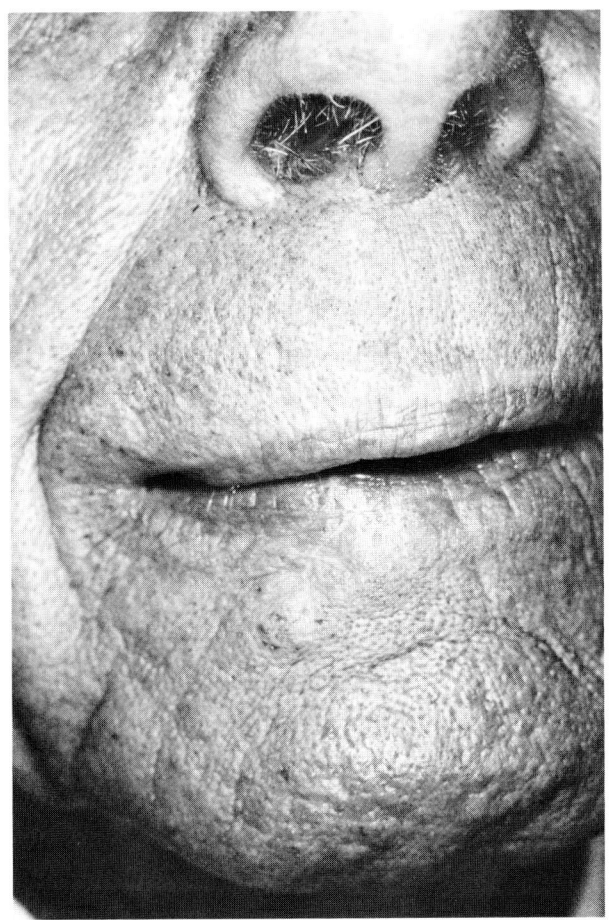

Figure 270. Appearance of the lip three months postoperatively showing slight erythema but excellent cosmetic results.

Figure 271. Planned excision of a recurrent basal cel carcinoma of the left lateral neck. (See Figures 272–274.)

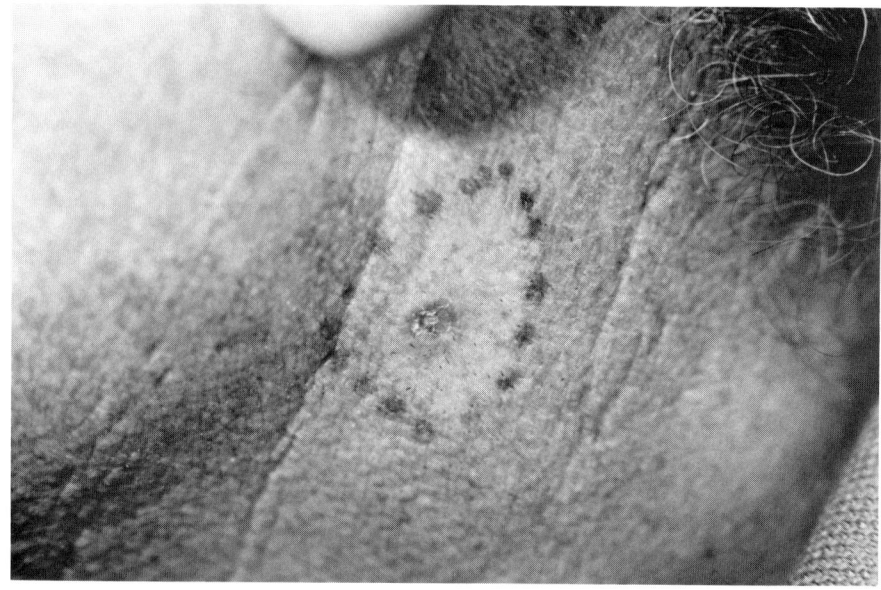

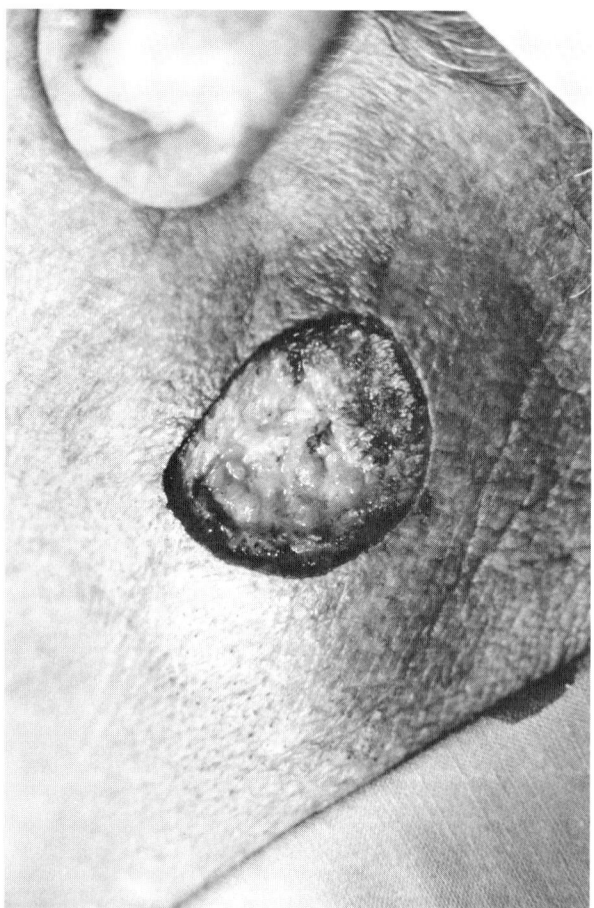

Figure 272. Appearance of the defect after the carbon dioxide laser has been used in its focused mode of operation to harvest the tissue in this anticoagulated patient.

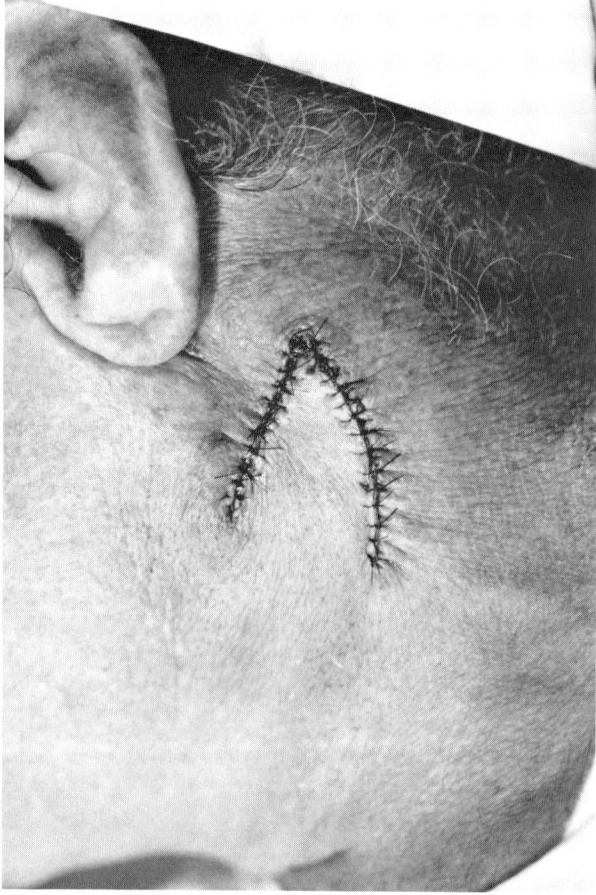

Figure 273. Once a tumor-free plane has been achieved, a small rotation flap is cut and mobilized with the focused carbon dioxide laser to permit primary repair of the wound.

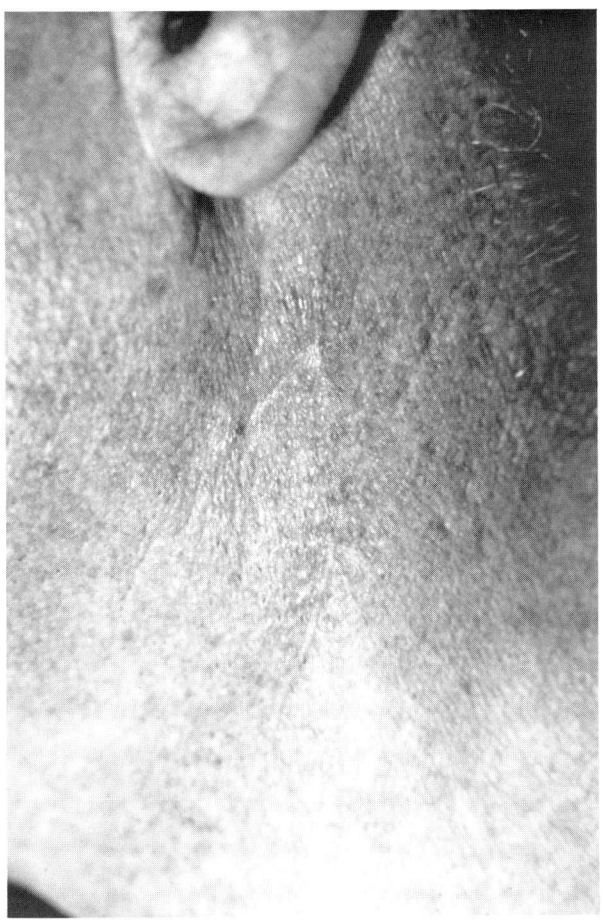

Figure 274. Appearance of the treatment site demonstrated in Figures 272 and 273 seen two months postoperatively.

BONE PERFORATION TO STIMULATE GRANULATION TISSUE

When an injury results in the exposure of cranial bone by the striping away of the periosteum, or if ablation of a cutaneous malignancy should result in exposure of cranial bone (Figure 275), granulation tissue will not grow over the exposed bone to bridge the defect with epithelium (Figure 276). A number of different techniques have been used in the past to stimulate the development of granulation tissue in these cases. The laser is one alternative method which permits this type of healing to occur.

Using the focused carbon dioxide laser beam of 0.1 mm diameter, 20 watts of power, and short pulses of 0.1 seconds, small holes can be created in the outer table of the cranium. This usually requires only one or two brief pulses of laser energy in order to perforate to the vascular diploe. When a small grid-like series of perforations has been created in an area of exposed cranial bone (Figure 277), granulation tissue will form through these small channels and allow the wound to heal by second intention (Figures 278–280). The main advantage of this technique is the speed with which it can be performed and the minimal trauma associated with its performance. However, it must be remembered that this technique should not be utilized in irradiated bone since the diploe may be avascular and direct perforation through the inner table of the skull may occur.

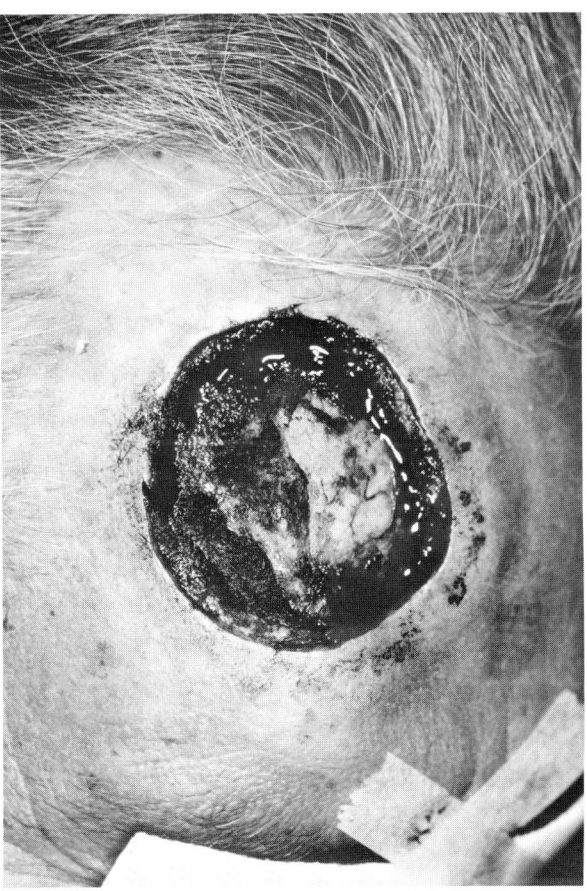

Figure 275. A large defect of the forehead showing exposure of the frontal bone due to basal cell carcinoma involvement of the periosteum.

134   Lasers in Skin Disease

Figure 276. Same patient seen in Figure 275 eight weeks after cancer treatment. The wound has failed to epithelialize across this portion of the exposed frontal bone.

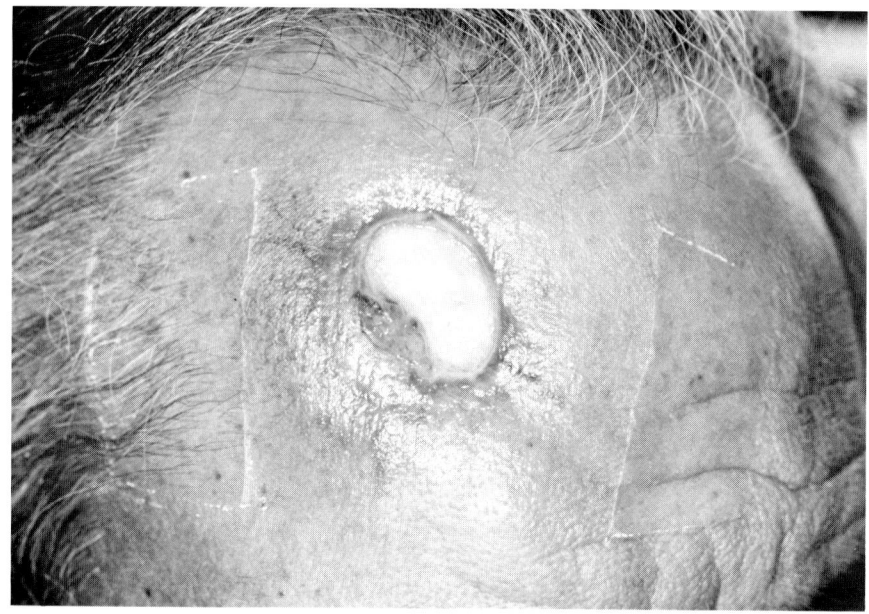

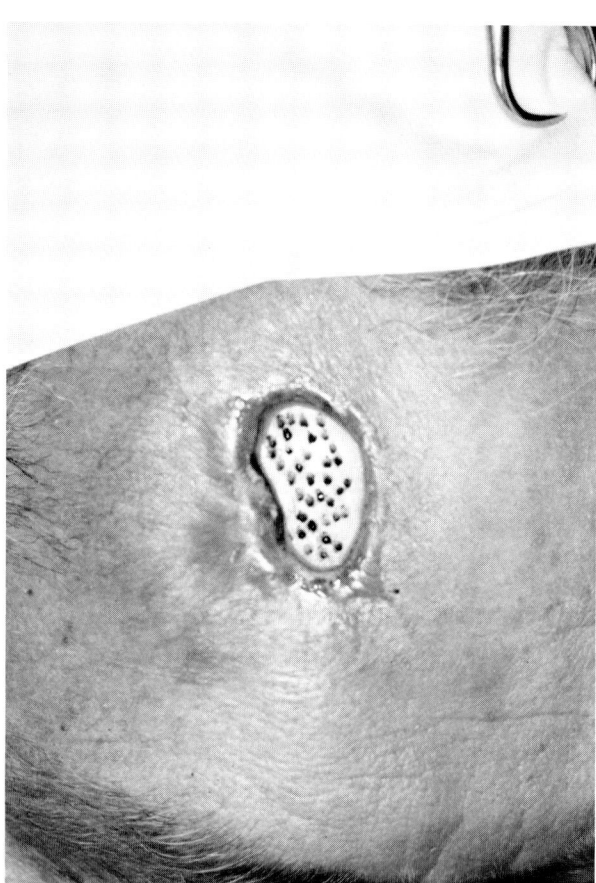

Figure 277. The appearance of the wound immediately after the carbon dioxide laser has been used in its focused mode of operation to create a series of small grid-like perforations through the outer table of the skull. (See Figures 275–280.)

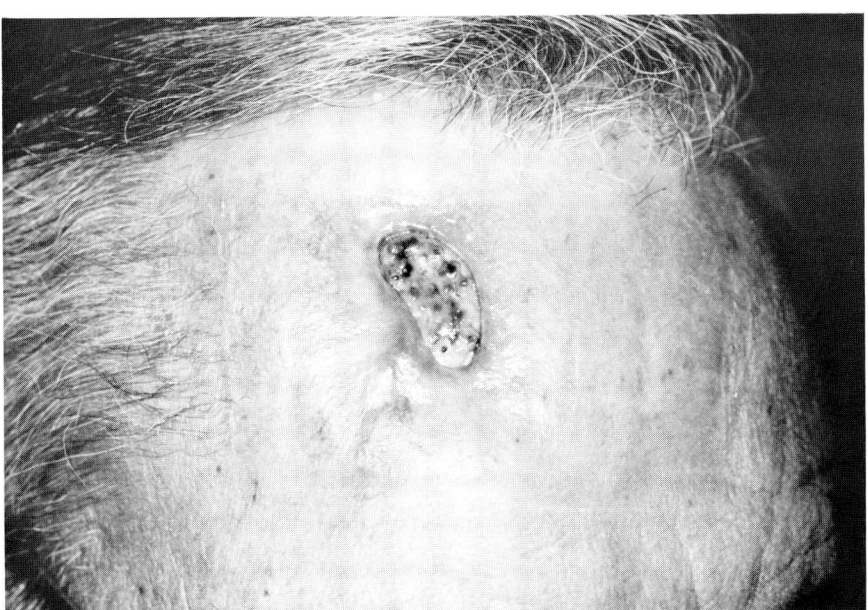

Figure 278. One week postoperatively, the patient shown in Figures 275–277 is starting to develop granulation tissue through the perforations created within the outer table of the skull.

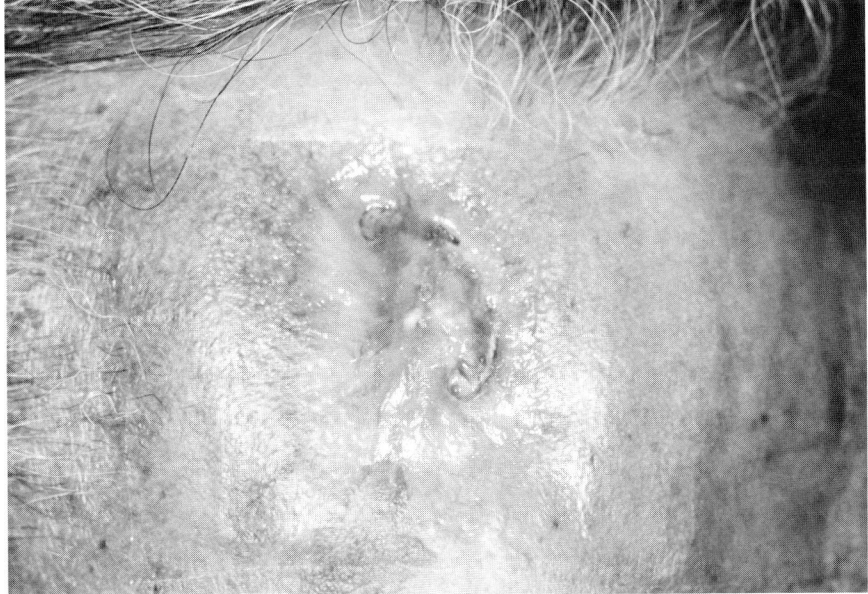

Figure 279. Clinical appearance of the healed wound six weeks after laser perforation of the outer table of the skull had been performed.

Figure 280. Final cosmetic result four months postoperatively showing a discernible scar but with supple skin and soft tissue bridging the defect shown initially in Figure 275.

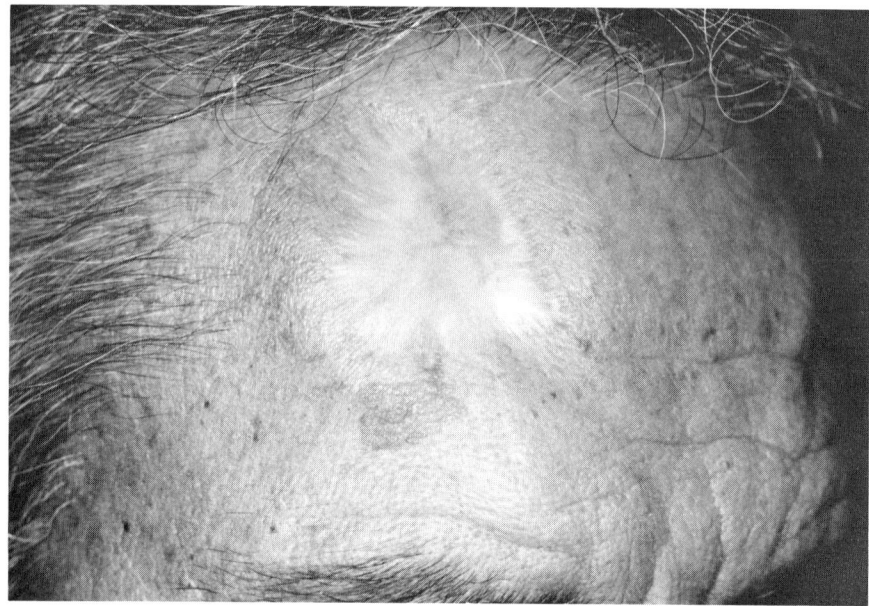

BIBLIOGRAPHY

Bailin PL, Ratz JL, Lutz-Nagey L: CO_2 laser modification of Mohs surgery. J Dermatol Surg Oncol 7:621–623, 1981.

Bailin PL, Wheeland RG: Carbon dioxide (CO_2) laser perforation of exposed cranial bone to stimulate granulation tissue. Plast Reconstr Surg 75:898–902, 1985.

David LM, Sanders G: CO_2 laser blepharoplasty: A comparison to cold steel and electrocautery. J Dermatol Surg Oncol 13:110–114, 1987.

Finsterbush A, Russo M, Ashur H: Healing and tensile strength of CO_2 laser incisions and scalpel wounds in rabbits. Plast Reconstr Surg 70:360–362, 1982.

Henderson DL, Crowwell TA, Mes LG: Argon and carbon dioxide laser treatment of hypertrophic and keloid scars. Lasers Surg Med 3:271–277, 1984.

Kantor GR, Wheeland RG, Bailin PL, et al: Treatment of earlobe keloids with carbon dioxide laser excision: A report of 16 cases. J Dermatol Surg Oncol 11:1063–1067, 1985.

Kantor GR, Ratz JL, Wheeland RG: Treatment of acne keloidalis nuchae with carbon dioxide laser. J Am Acad Dermatol 14:263–267, 1986.

Kirschner RA: Cutaneous plastic surgery with the CO_2 laser. Surg Clin North Am 64:871–883, 1984.

Norris CW, Mullarky MB: Experimental skin incision made with the carbon dioxide laser. Laryngoscope 92:416–419, 1982.

Sacchini V, Lovo GF, Arioli N, et al: Carbon dioxide laser in scalp tumor surgery. Laser Surg Med 4:261–269, 1984.

Slutzki S, Shafir R, Bornstein LA: Use of the carbon dioxide laser for large excisions with minimal blood loss. Plast Reconstr Surg 60:250–255, 1977.

Wheeland RG, Bailin PL: Scalp reduction surgery with the carbon dioxide laser. J Dermatol Surg Oncol 10:565–569, 1984.

Wheeland RG, Bailin PL, Ratz JL: Combined carbon dioxide laser excision and vaporization in the treatment of rhinophyma. J Dermatol Surg Oncol 13:172–177, 1987.

6 Future Applications of Lasers in Cutaneous Disease

In the nearly 26 years since the original development of the first laser, many remarkable changes have occurred. It seems obvious that in the near future, a variety of new laser systems will be developed that will allow physicians to more effectively treat a large number of cutaneous lesions of the hand and neck for which now no successful form of therapy exists. While the carbon dioxide and argon lasers offer us significantly useful tools in the management of many different conditions, there is no doubt that additional changes are expected. A review of some of the lasers that are currently available, but that so far have proven to have only limited usefulness in the treatment of cutaneous disorders will be given.

Nd:YAG

The neodymium-YAG (yttrium-aluminum-garnet) laser is a near infrared laser light source of 1,060 mm. This laser—unlike the energy of the argon laser which is absorbed by chromophores of the skin or the energy of the carbon dioxide laser which is absorbed by water—is absorbed by protein. As a consequence of this, when energy from this laser impacts tissue, it is scattered significantly and causes a diffuse thermal effect. As a consequence, this laser is relatively imprecise and can cause a zonal type of destruction much larger than is clinically apparent. This laser is, however, extremely effective in providing hemostasis and has been used extensively in gastroenterology and neurosurgery.

Recent research studies have shown that the Nd:YAG laser can cause inhibition of fibroblasts in tissue culture. For this reason, this laser may prove to be useful in the treatment of a number of fibrotic diseases, such as keloids. Also, the Nd:YAG laser has been used effectively to treat deeply located angiomas or angiomas with large vascular channels since it penetrates deeper into tissue than the argon laser. One technique that has been used to improve its effect on large vessels is to compress the boggy angioma first with a glass or plastic slide and deliver the Nd:YAG laser energy through the plastic or glass to the dilated vessels.

Laser welding of incisions of the skin has also been investigated using the Nd:YAG laser with low irradiance. It appears that while other lasers are also capable of producing a protein coagulum and of sealing incised wounds, the Nd:YAG laser may be effectively used in the future to precisely reanastomose small vascular channels, nerves, and organs of reproduction. How useful this proves to be remains largely unanswered at this time.

TUNABLE DYE LASERS

The tunable dye laser is an interesting instrument since it can be adjusted over a spectrum of different wavelengths to emit light energy of different colors. The current technology allows dye laser energy, using various organic compounds, to be adjusted from 488 to 638 nm. These lasers, which are extremely expensive to purchase, can produce laser light of blue, yellow, orange, and red color. Each of these different wavelengths of light can be expected to have different effects on tissue, so the dye laser is extremely versatile. Yellow light, of 577 nm, has been used extensively in the treatment of vascular conditions. This wavelength appears to be more selective in its effects on the vascular tissue than argon laser energy since its emission more closely parallels the beta absorption peak for hemoglobin. This specificity of interaction allows minimal injury to surrounding tissue and yet maximizes thermal injury to vascular spaces.

The red wavelength of the dye laser (633 nm) or gold head vapor laser (630 nm) is being used now in the treatment of refractory cutaneous neoplasms in a procedure known as photodynamic therapy (PDT). This technique employs the intravenous injection of a photoactive chemical, dihematoporphyrin ether. Two to three days after this material has been injected, the tumor is irradiated using the red light of the dye laser. The photosensitive chemical is transformed through the interaction of this wavelength of light energy and results in the formation of a singlet oxygen radical which causes oxidation of various components of the cell, producing cell death.

The main benefits of photodynamic therapy includes minimal injury to surrounding normal tissue and that it can be performed in patients who have undergone prior radiotherapy or chemotherapy. The main disadvantage of this technique is that the red wavelength of light used to create this photosensitive reaction in tissue is relatively nonpenetrating and thus, for thick cancers, an incomplete or partial response may be obtained. Also, there is a persistent difficulty for the patient with diffuse photosensitivity which may last for several months. Additional experience with tumors of the head and neck using this modality are underway.

One other laser source is capable of delivering energy of red color wavelength of 630 nm for the photosensitivity reaction of PDT to occur. This source of laser energy is the gold head vapor laser. This extremely experimental and expensive instrument has been utilized to produce light of proper wavelength for this technique, but its availability is limited and only minimal experience with this laser technique has been published at this time.

EXCIMER LASER

Excimer stands for *exci*ted di*mer*. This laser is a relatively new addition to laser technology. These lasers, which emit in the ultraviolet range of the electromagnetic spectrum, are capable of delivering extremely short (nanosecond) pulses of ultraviolet energy to tissue. This delivery permits very precise thermal effects without injury to adjacent tissue or even organelles of a single cell. An example of how this laser can be used is the technical possibility of limiting injury to just the melanosomes within a cell of the skin without damage to other vital subcellular parts. This phe-

nomenon is known as selective photothermolysis. This is an exciting area of much current research and it may change our ability to treat a variety of diseases in the not too distant future.

COPPER VAPOR LASER

The copper vapor laser is another current investigational tool that can deliver a variety of different wavelengths: 510, 540, 577, 620, 650 and 690 nm. At the present time it is typically used to produce yellow light of 577 nm and is employed to treat vascular lesions of the skin, much as the dye laser is used. Additional research in this area will be required before this instrument becomes widely available as a clinical tool.

HELIUM-NEON (HeNe) LASER

While the helium-neon laser is certainly not a new laser system, recent studies have shown that this laser, of wavelength 633 nm, can stimulate collagen production by fibroblasts in culture. Whether this laser could be used as a form of biostimulation for healing of some cutaneous wounds remains in some doubt. However, additional research in this area is currently underway and should resolve this controversy.

BIBLIOGRAPHY

Abergel RP, Meeker CA, Dwyer RM, et al: Nonthermal effects of Nd:YAG laser on biological functions of human skin fibroblasts in culture. Lasers Surg Med 3:279–284, 1984.

Abergel R, Meeker C, Lam T, et al: Control of connective tissue metabolism by lasers: Recent developments and future prospects. J Am Acad Dermatol 11:1142–1150, 1984.

Abergel RP, Lyons RD, Castel JC, et al: Biostimulation of wound healing by lasers: Experimental approaches in animal models and in fibroblast cultures. J Dermatol Surg Oncol 13:127–133, 1987.

Anderson RR, Parrish JA: Selective photothermolysis: Precise microsurgery by selective absorption of pulsed radiation. Science 220:524–527, 1983.

Anderson RR, Jaenicke KF, Parrish JA: Mechanisms of selective vascular changes caused by dye lasers. Lasers Surg Med 3:211–215, 1983.

Berns MW: Preface: Hematoporphyrin derivative photoradiation therapy. Lasers Surg Med 4:1–4, 1984.

Brunner R, Landthaler M, Haina D, et al: Treatment of

benign, semi-malignant, and malignant skin tumors with the Nd:YAG laser. Lasers Surg Med 5:105–110, 1985.

Garden JM, Tan OT, Parrish JA: The pulsed dye laser: Its use at 577 nm wavelength. J Dermatol Surg Oncol 13:134–138, 1987.

Goldman L, Gregory RO, LaPlant M: Preliminary investigative studies with PDT in dermatologic and plastic surgery. Lasers Surg Med 5:453–456, 1986.

Goldman L, Taylor A, Putnam T: New developments with the heavy metal vapor lasers for the dermatologist. J Dermatol Surg Oncol 13:163–165, 1987.

McCaughan JS Jr, Guy JT, Hawley P, et al: Hematoporphyrin–derivative and photoradiation therapy of malignant tumors. Lasers Surg Med 3:199–209, 1983.

Wile AG, Coffey J, Nahabedian MY, et al: Laser photoradiation therapy of cancer. Lasers Surg Med 4:5–12, 1984.

Index